We're in crisis. Abandoning our ancient commitment to character, to integrity of soul, we are being ravaged from the inside. These pages, from such a wise, heart-full guide, are truths to heed if we want to be whole. Chuck is a beloved professor and therapist—but more, he's a friend committed to loving well and telling the truth. And God knows, we sure need the truth right now. This is a book for our disintegrating time.

WINN COLLIER, director of the Eugene Peterson Center for Christian Imagination and author of *Love Big, Be Well* and *A Burning in My Bones: The Authorized Biography of Eugene H. Peterson*

Chuck DeGroat is a soul cardiologist, a wise, kind, and brilliant reader of the human heart. He surgically engages one of the key issues of our era: character. Many have eschewed character for power, notoriety, and disparagement of those who differ from us. This compelling, beautifully written book calls us to become who we, at our best, long to be. Chuck not only helps us envision the glory of a good character, but he also provides clarity about the practices, conversations, and reflection needed to be a presence that manifests the face of God. You are about to embark on a journey that will restore your heart.

DAN B. ALLENDER, PHD, professor of counseling psychology, founding president, The Seattle School of Theology and Psychology

In the midst of our unmoored, image-obsessed culture, Dr. Chuck DeGroat offers us the grounding wisdom we so often forget: God is with us as we become ourselves. With kindness and deft insight, DeGroat leads us through the practical, courageous, and often slow work required to cultivate maturity and true character. In so doing, *Who You're Becoming* serves as a powerful and needed guide for anyone wanting to go beyond a try-hard faith or mere surface-level change—so they can deepen into their truest, beloved selves.

AUNDI KOLBER, MA, LPC, therapist and author of *Try Softer* and *Strong like Water*

Rarely do I refer to a book as a "must read." But rarely do I come across a book as incisive and inspiring as this one. It is indeed a "must read" for anyone taking up the mantle of ministry and leadership. With timeless truths spoken directly to our particular age, Chuck has given us a great gift in this remarkable and healing book.

AMANDA HELD OPELT, author of *Holy Unhappiness*

At our best and truest we are pilgrims, called into lifelong journeys, which are "cultivated through faith, strengthened through hope, and embodied through love." In his deeply imagined new book, it is clear that Chuck DeGroat is a true doctor of the soul, paying attention to what matters most in our desire for a coherence born of the reordering of our loves and longings. Drawing us into a prayerful examination of our selves, always both honest and yet hopeful, with his poetic blessing we are invited to ponder more carefully and to live more faithfully. Threaded through with the wisdom of church history and the insight of contemporary science, in their different ways addressing our disposition to fragmentation and our yearning for integration, *Who You're Becoming* should find its way into conversations and classrooms the world over—with sons of Adam and daughters of Eve who are becoming more whole people, and therefore more holy people.

STEVEN GARBER, author of *Hints of Hope: Essays on Making Peace with the Proximate* and Senior Fellow for Vocation and the Common Good, the M.J. Murdock Charitable Trust

Chuck has written a book that should immediately be required reading for all of us, whether we are in formal leadership or not; while character should be our shared concern, we are constantly being tempted to focus on presentation instead. He therefore asks us fair but too often ignored questions, helps us distinguish between personality and character, provides ample wisdom, and consistently points us toward healthy formation that pushes against fragmentation and instead toward wholeness. Please read it slowly and with the courage it requires so that you might experience the hope it promises.

KELLY M. KAPIC, author of *You're Only Human* and *Christian Life*

Character is not curated. It is cultivated. The gift Chuck gives us in this book is the wisdom of a quarter century as therapist, pastor, and professor. *Who You're Becoming* refuses performative authenticity and the fauxnerability that too often passes for Christian maturity. In their place, Chuck offers the slow ripening of the soul moved from survival to connection, from disorder to devotion, from charisma to character. Drawing on Scripture and the wisdom of the Christian tradition, he answers the crisis of character in our narcissistic age with the patient kindness of God. I need this book. So does every leader weary of the masks.

JUSTIN S. HOLCOMB, Episcopal bishop, seminary professor, and author of *Rid of My Disgrace*

In this beautiful invitation to courageous wholeheartedness, *Who You're Becoming* is a gentle and grounded companion on the journey of change. Weaving together a pastoral heart, therapeutic insight, and anchored hope, Chuck lights the way for a compelling and compassionate exploration of who we long to be, and how we long to live.

LAURA THIEN, MSW, LISW-CP, therapist and executive director of GRACE

In *Who You're Becoming*, Chuck DeGroat reclaims the lost territory of character formation and shows us a fresh path through an understanding of our nervous system response. Chuck invites us on an exploratory journey, linking our character to our unhealthy patterns of self-protection and disconnection. And of course Chuck invites us into the slow, courageous, and essential work of integration so that the deepest parts of our souls can relax into the love of God. Chuck's writings have been essential reading in my life for almost a decade, and this book is now top of my recommendation list.

STEVE CUSS, pastor and author

Chuck DeGroat has written a wise and searching book for a moment when too many leaders have been formed for visibility but not for trustworthiness. *Who You're Becoming* offers a penetrating, deeply humane, and spiritually serious vision of character formation that joins theology, psychology, and the slow work of grace in ways that many leaders badly need. I will recommend this book to my clients with enthusiasm and deep appreciation.

TOD BOLSINGER, AE Sloan Leadership, author of *Canoeing the Mountains* and the Practicing Change Series

We are living in a moment of profound and painful unveiling, and this labor of love is a gift for such a time as this. With hard-won, embodied wisdom, Chuck locates the truths of modern psychology inside the ancient systems of spiritual formation, calling us beyond the performative and into the deep waters where true character is slowly, courageously and intentionally forged. This is a book that holds a mirror to our current age, and invites us into the long journey from fragmentation to wholeness and from nervous system reactivity into being rooted and grounded in love. Chuck so generously weaves together insights, stories, resources, reflection questions, and practices to help us locate ourselves in these pages, drawing us toward a wholeness and belonging we are meant for and will need in order to resist the perils of this day. He invites us to know even more the God of love who is tending to the restoration of all things. Thank you feels wildly insufficient.

RACHAEL CLINTON CHEN, trauma practitioner and pastoral leader with The Allender Center at The Seattle School of Theology and Psychology

Many approaches to cultivating Christian character remain curiously disembodied, overlooking how our nervous systems and hidden patterns can quietly subvert our best intentions. In this illuminating work, Chuck DeGroat brings these often-ignored dimensions into the light, drawing on decades of experience as a counselor and the wisdom of a seasoned pastoral theologian. In an age marked by restless striving and spiritual adolescence, this book offers a surprising and beautiful recovery of a slower, truer path—one that leads us to become "rooted and grounded in love" (Ephesians 3:17). A gem of a book—one to savor, and to revisit.

J. TODD BILLINGS, author of *The End of the Christian Life: How Embracing Our Mortality Frees Us to Truly Live*

At a time when therapeutic language has become social currency and character formation has become a product rather than a practice, Chuck DeGroat calls us back to the slow, unglamorous, embodied work of actually becoming someone. Drawing on neuroscience, ancient Christian wisdom, and a keen eye for the performance culture of our time, this book refuses every shortcut and offers something rarer than technique: a genuinely integrated vision of what human transformation looks like. What distinguishes this book is that it was written by someone whose life bears witness to everything in it.

ELIZABETH PENNOCK, PHD, LPC, associate professor of counseling, director of MA in clinical mental health counseling program, Western Theological Seminary

Chuck DeGroat's latest book, *Who You're Becoming*, is a powerful and much-needed invitation to the slow, sacred work of becoming a whole person. In a world that rewards image over integrity and platform over character, this message could not be more timely. What makes this book especially compelling is that Chuck doesn't just write about this kind of inner formation—he embodies it. Chuck is a person of deep integrity, humility, and courageous self-awareness, and that is exactly why his is a voice we can trust—and why this is a book every single one of us needs to read.

DR. ALISON COOK, author of *The Secure Soul* and host of *The Best of You* podcast who you're becoming

CHUCK DEGROAT

who you're becoming

THE SLOW AND COURAGEOUS WORK OF CULTIVATING CHARACTER IN A NARCISSISTIC AGE

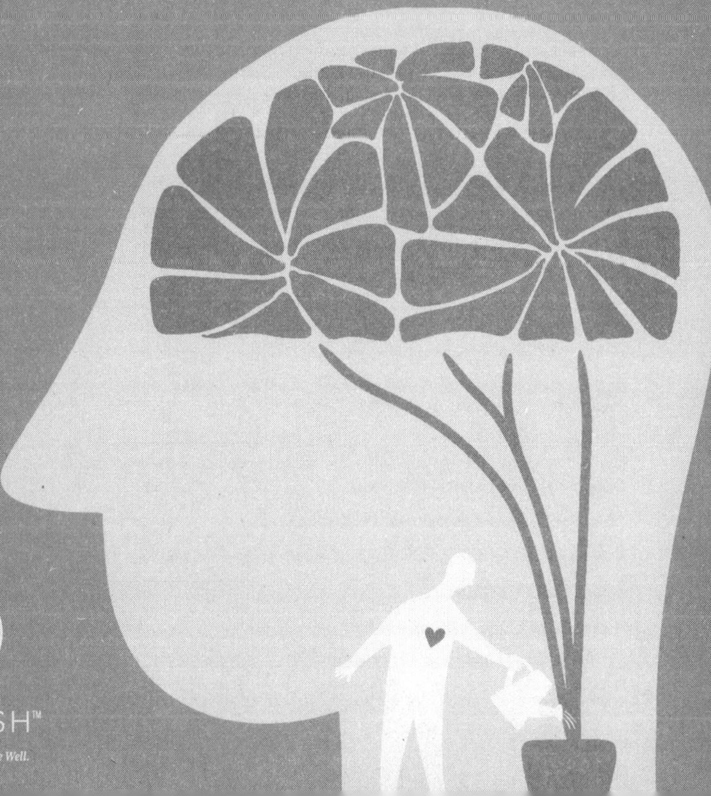

TYNDALE
REFRESH™
Think Well. Live Well. Be Well.

Visit Tyndale online at tyndale.com.

Visit Chuck at chuckdegroat.net.

Who You're Becoming: The Slow and Courageous Work of Cultivating Character in a Narcissistic Age

Cover design by Dean H. Renninger

Interior design by Brandi Davis

Published in association with Don Gates of the literary agency The Gates Group; www.the-gates-group.com.

For information about special discounts for bulk purchases, please contact Tyndale House Publishers at csresponse@tyndale.com, or call 1-855-277-9400.

The case examples in this book are fictional composites based on the author's professional interactions with hundreds of clients over the years. All names are invented, and any resemblance between these fictional characters and real people is coincidental.

Library of Congress Cataloging-in-Publication Data

A catalog record for this book is available from the Library of Congress.

ISBN 978-1-4964-8318-8

Printed in the United States of America

32 31 30 29 28 27 26
7 6 5 4 3 2 1

contents

INTRODUCTION

can I trust you?

We often tend to select leaders in the Christian world according to their gifts rather than their character. . . . Spiritual maturity is measured by character, by the fruit of the Spirit of God in a life.
DIANE LANGBERG

Woe to you, teachers of the law and Pharisees, you hypocrites! You clean the outside of the cup and dish, but inside they are full of greed and self-indulgence.
MATTHEW 23:25

I stood beside him in the church choir.

Months later, he was arrested for murder.

Back then, he seemed like the kind of man no one would ever question—steady, respected, a pillar of our community.

Sure, he seemed a little aloof during choir practice, but I was just a teenager, not noteworthy to someone so respected. Sure, he lacked a little warmth, but I knew he had a reputation of being a loving husband and a good father.

Each emerging detail of the twisted tale—how he shot and strangled his wife amidst an affair—rocked our community and rattled me, leaving me with lingering questions. How could I reconcile the man I thought I knew with the man he really was? How could a man of apparent character hold such contradictions? If he could do this, could I trust other leaders?

I had thought of him as one of my heroes: Jean Vanier, founder of L'Arche, a community in Trosly-Breuil in northern France founded to dignify women and men with disabilities. My first church office as a pastor in the late 1990s featured photographed images of several of my heroes, his face among them.

Vanier's ministry and character inspired me—his kind smile and gentle presence evident in every image and recording of him. Sometimes I'd watch his moving YouTube videos just to remind myself that there are profoundly good leaders—and profoundly good human beings—out there. Vanier's person and work would later become the defining feature of a seminary class I taught, a course I hoped would inspire another generation of kind and generous pastors.

But a few years after teaching that course, just as the world was gripped by the news of a growing pandemic, I received the kind of text I dread.

Vanier had engaged in sexual misconduct.

And not just once. An independent 2023 report would find that Vanier engaged in manipulative and coercive sexual relationships with at least twenty-five adult women under his spiritual direction. The relationships involved spiritual and psychological coercion, with Vanier justifying sexual acts using mystical and theological language to portray them as a form of divine connection.[1]

This wasn't a self-serving minister or a calculating politician, but a man universally revered as a living saint. He was a mentor to the late

Henri Nouwen, whose quiet devotion to the disability community seemed untouched by a need for recognition.

Many within the Christian community were left with heavy questions: If Vanier can't be trusted, who can? How can we ever really know what's true? How do we make sense of it all?

In 2008, our family moved cross-country so I could join the staff of a thriving center-city church. Within two years, I helped launch a counseling center, a fellows program, and a missional training center—all the while teaching, counseling, and occasionally preaching.

The subtle signs of burnout became more obvious—stomach pain, sleeplessness, too much coffee to start the day and too much alcohol to finish it. During a silent retreat I was leading at a conference center, a colleague and I snuck out for a lavish meal and enough drink to leave me fuzzy and faltering as I led the next morning's session.

But awareness of my own contradictions wasn't enough. It would take another year or two and a sudden and serious hospitalization to awaken me. What should have been a straightforward gallbladder removal surgery revealed something worse—my system was septic, the toll of my own trauma and fragmentation.

How can the pursuit even of good things blind us to our character contradictions?

The Crisis of Character

I don't know the specifics of the story you're bringing to these pages, but I do know you're bringing one.

Maybe you bear the confusion of the incongruity you see and hear about each day. The neighbor down the block who kept to himself, suddenly arrested on charges of child pornography. The trusted elementary school principal, now fired for misconduct. The family doctor, who faithfully helped your children through ear infections, caught prescribing controlled substances to minors. The popular pastor of a growing and influential church revealed to be a serial adulterer.

With each revelation, you ask again: *Who can I trust?*

But after that whisper of a question, if you listen closely enough, you might begin to hear another: *What happens when* I'm *called to account?*

After all, you have your own contradictions too.

You long to live with Christlike character, but you're also aware of how you lose your temper, how you secretly judge people, how your eyes linger a little longer than they should. You silently wonder if you're capable of some significant moral compromise. Perhaps seeing the salacious stories, you quietly whisper to yourself, "There but for the grace of God go I."

From the fractured trust in the highest political, corporate, and ecclesial offices in the land to the fragmented places in our own hearts, we're facing a profound unveiling.

And what's been uncovered is not just an individual crisis but a systemic one. In my work as a therapist, pastor, professor, and consultant, including more than twenty-five years in the spiritual abuse space, I've noted a profound cultural shift: Qualities of charisma, charm, credentials, confidence, and skilled communication are being elevated at the cost of character.

So much has become *performative*: Behaviors or expressions seem to signal virtue, expertise, alignment, or authenticity, but they lack genuine depth, substance, or integrity. They are done in the name of image management rather than deep formation. Metrics, branding, and platform have become benchmarks of success that must be constantly and rigorously curated. We are increasingly driven by external validation (what others think, say, or reward) rather than our own internal convictions and personal integrity. We feel immense pressure to immediately respond to complex social issues, to side publicly in disembodied disputes, to quickly signal concern for global injustices instead of engaging in difficult, long-term local work. The temptation to posture rather than to pause—to be *seen* as righteous rather than to *pursue* what is right—can feel unbearably strong.

Spiritual growth is reduced to informational note-taking and sermon-spectating under bright lights and from big personalities, trading intentional formation for a kind of ecclesial voyeurism. Embodied relational, liturgical, and confessional pathways of growth and discipleship are exchanged for a drive-through spirituality that fills the belly but fails to nurture the soul.

In recent years a further complication has emerged: the new cultural embrace of therapeutic language and theories. What once was a pervasive suspicion of psychology and therapy, particularly in ecclesial spaces, has turned into a performative embrace. Those who've mastered the language of health or awareness can readily name the books they've consulted and the tools they claim to have incorporated into their relational and spiritual practices; it can be deeply confusing and traumatizing when these same practitioners harm others, perhaps even using the very resources created to cultivate health.

It feels bleak because it is. We have more insights and resources than ever for emotional and spiritual health, but it seems that they've not reached the depths of our hearts—where character is formed.

We're becoming shaped more by perception than presence, more by applause than authenticity; this is narcissism's new face in a digital age.

The Courage to Name What's True

This is the reckoning: a painful but necessary confrontation with all the ways we've traded true character for charisma, formation for information, communion for control, discipleship for display, transformation for techniques.

We cannot paper over this crisis with platitudes, quick fixes, or superficial reforms. The way forward cannot be reactive or cosmetic. It must be a wholesale reformation, a ground-up reconstruction, a reintegration of what has been fragmented, distorted, and disguised.

As the late author and religious scholar Phyllis Tickle wrote, "About every five hundred years the empowered structures of institutionalized Christianity, whatever they may be at that time, become an intolerable carapace that must be shattered in order that renewal and new growth may occur." Tickle credits this idea to the Right Reverend Mark Dyer, Anglican bishop, who refers to this as the "giant rummage sale."[2]

For many people, the language of character may feel outdated today, overshadowed by talk of competency, health, emotional intelligence, or even spiritual formation. Others will affirm that character still matters, but their solution to the crisis in character is to focus on simple remedies. However, character formation isn't about minor modifications—a new breathing practice, a short sabbatical, a few books on spiritual growth on your side table.

This is not about retrofitting old structures but dismantling what no longer serves and rebuilding on foundations that can endure—as reformations have done before. If we are to see a recovery of trust and integrity, it will demand a radical reorientation in how we form leaders, how we imagine success, and how we live our lives before God and one another.

In short, it's time to cultivate the courage to tell the truth about who we are and who we've become. It's time to embrace the slow, costly work of character formation.

But what is character? And how is it developed?

A Course in Character Formation

Character is revealed over time through the habits of the heart and the choices that emerge naturally from deeply rooted convictions rather than the whims of circumstance. Its understated and steady presence—seen in the quiet courage to tell the truth, the humility to admit fault, the consistency of integrity over time, and the ability to hold power without using it to harm—may be undervalued in a world that embraces the sparkle and grandiosity of charisma and credentials.

While charm and expertise have their place, I sense the need to shift our imaginations toward more substantial pathways that lead to character change. The beatitudes offer us a compelling vision (Matthew 5:1-12). These are not mere moral benchmarks or abstract blessings but descriptions of the *flourishing life*—the kind that aligns with God's Kingdom and leads to wholeness. "Blessed are . . ." is best translated as "Flourishing are . . ." to emphasize that Jesus offers a vision of the good life, a life of character shaped by humility, mercy, wholeness, and peacemaking.[3] In this view, the beatitudes are formative—they describe the kind of person whose inner life and outer relationships reflect deep congruence with the heart of God. They invite us to become who we are, at our core, as image bearers created for worth, belonging, and purpose in the world.

And of course, Jesus sums up the entire law and prophets in two commands: "Love the Lord your God with all your heart and with all your soul and with all your mind. . . . Love your neighbor as yourself" (Matthew 22:37, 39). This reveals the *telos*—the ultimate objective—of character: *love*. Not love as sentiment, but love as self-giving, shalom-seeking, justice-making, relational wholeness. Mature character, in other words, is not defined by public posture or performance but by one's capacity to love wisely, courageously, and sacrificially. The apostle Paul encourages us to aim for lives that exemplify the fruit of the Spirit—a full expression of love that is accompanied by joy, peace, patience, kindness, goodness, faithfulness, gentleness, and self-control (Galatians 5:22-23).

If personality is how we show up—funny, shy, pensive, charming, bold, sarcastic, reserved, talkative, intense, magnetic, awkward, or agreeable—*character* suggests something more substantial and enduring: our deep-seated dispositions, consistent traits, embedded habits, even our chronic behaviors. Imagine a sculptor carving an image into stone or a metalworker imprinting an image onto a coin. Imagine the deep, permanent grooves that hold up amidst life's changing weather patterns.

Thus, character is the slow-formed architecture that shapes our consistent choices so that we can live in alignment with love. It reflects our capacity for inner integration—of our desires, wounds, and fears. When we are able to acknowledge and reconcile the internal patterns and motives that drive our behavior and emotions, our outer life increasingly flows from wholeness rather than compulsion.

This is evidence of an inner life reordered for the sake of embodied love.

In a world where personality pops, fauxnerability fools, and power platforms, we must be courageous enough to subversively dig deep and pursue grounded, mature, and transformed lives. The temptation to perform is strong. But the invitation of Christ is deeper—not to perform, but to become ourselves. Not to signal virtue, but to live with integrity. Not to be admired, but to be whole.

This is the journey I want to invite you on. As we grow into the kind of person whose inner life embodies love, power, and presence with integrity, we'll develop pathways not just for better health, but for deep change.

We'll do this in three parts.

Part 1 explores the *foundation* of character development. Schools and businesses have developed entire programs to encourage students and workers to treat one another with courtesy and civility. And Sunday school classes train children to live righteously. These programs have their place, and much that has been written on character speaks to behaving and acting the right way. Yet I'll ask a more fundamental question: What are the inner conditions necessary for deep transformation? While I'm all for behavior change, we've got to resist the impulse toward quick comebacks and cosmetic alterations that shortcut real, substantial change. Instead, we'll consider how to reenvision transformative change as something that must begin much deeper—at the neurobiological level.

Part 2 explores the *maturation* of character. If the architecture of our character is shaped from our first days and years, we need to think clearly and carefully about how character deepens and matures—in parenting, in church formation processes, in educational spaces, in time-honored initiatory practices. In these chapters, we'll hear from ancient and contemporary Christian guides who offer maps we might follow on the transformative journey. And we'll also discover a surprising but significant twist on the old adage that suffering forms character.

Part 3 explores the *transformation* that enables us to live with faith, hope, and love—which is to say, to live renewed, resilient, and relationally trustworthy lives. Character change is revealed not in short-term tweaks but in long-term consistency as we become more grounded, expectant, and attuned. In the final chapter, we'll see how character is lived out within complex relational systems where, without the foundational work of part 1, our anxiety might not only impact others but harm them. Yet we'll see how, once we engage in the foundational work and maturation process, our presence has the power to transform.

The story of character formation I want to tell you doesn't pit Scripture against psychology, ancient virtue ethics against neuroscience, or sin against styles of coping. No, we need it all today. We need the philosophers and the poets, the theologians and the therapists. They'll all find a voice in the chapters to come.

The Hope of This Work

Almost fifteen years ago, I consulted in a painful church situation that involved an extramarital affair between a pastor and a staff member. The pastor's attempt at a cover-up and his failure to disclose his mistakes, even when confronted, led to further pain and harm for the woman whose trust he exploited, for the wife he betrayed, for the congregation he deceived.

To my shock, the leadership of the church took their beloved pastor's sin seriously, both as a moral failure and as an abuse of power. They committed resources, not just to their own restoration and health, but to the long-term rehabilitation and health of the survivor, the (now-fired) pastor, and his spouse. The survivor felt seen, heard, and honored, and the church followed through on their rehabilitation plan for years after.

I tracked the process for some time with hope and gratitude. But after a decade I lost connection. And then I ran into the pastor on a street corner in a city I was visiting. I asked how he was doing, and he took a few minutes to describe a process that involved reparation, counseling, challenging marital work, a reimagined vocation, and long-term healing. He seemed genuinely well.

"Chuck, you told me it'd be at least ten years before you'd ever consider letting me transition back into church work, and it's about that time—so I've applied for a church job," he said.

For the first time, I grew a bit anxious. But I listened closely.

"I've applied to be the site manager of a Presbyterian church in town," he said. "Basically, that means cleaning toilets and changing lightbulbs."

He laughed. And I followed.

"My wife and I talk about one day finding our way back into pastoral ministry, but I've discovered this is slow work. And I like how this steady and slow progress feels. It's much better than the awful and stressful pace I'd gone at before."

With that, he told me that he could hardly wait to serve the church again, one toilet at a time. In him, I saw a man who'd left the masks behind and was becoming who he is at his core.

This is how the tree trunk of character thickens—ring by quiet ring. Not with the rapid upward stretch of ambition, but with the slow growth of repentance, reflection, and repair. The outer bark may look unchanging to passersby, but beneath the surface, the core is forming anew—denser, steadier, stronger—the hidden evidence of character change. This pastor's story is a witness to the slow, subterranean grace of healing overflowing into outward fruit. What was once hollowed out by secrecy and shame has been refilled by honesty and humility.

This is the kind of growth we need more of—slow, hidden, rooted.

Less platform and more presence.

Fewer quick fixes and more deep transformation.

There are no shortcuts to this kind of fruitful life and Christlike character. It's not something that can be crowdsourced or curated, simply tweaked with a few spiritual practices, a season of self-care, or a book on your personality type. We must reimagine spiritual growth, not as the means of acquiring information or mastering techniques, but as a lifelong movement into depth and integrity, cultivated through faith, strengthened through hope, and embodied through love. It is nurtured in the quiet, often unseen spaces where no one is watching, where the Spirit meets us, not on stage, but in the shadows. It is forged slowly—measured not in weeks, but in years. Sometimes decades.

The Spirit does not rush nor relent. In hidden places, in quiet lives, in small acts of courage and truth-telling, the Spirit is already at work—deepening roots, strengthening trunks, preparing us to bear the fruit of a renewed and resilient character.

My friends, I know what I'm asking of you. I know what I'm asking of myself. It won't be easy, but it will be sacred. The reckoning will bear fruit. I'm convinced of it because I trust the Spirit who hovers over chaos, who broods over what is formless and void, who brings life out of death and calls forth beauty from broken places.

I long for this to be a resource for all who wrestle as I do, who are weary but hungry for hope and longing to trust. Hope doesn't erase the mess or stitch together the fractures overnight. Real hope, as you'll see, grows in quieter places—beneath the noise, beneath our striving, beneath the temptation to manage appearances. It emerges slowly, often imperceptibly, in the small acts of truth-telling, the humble confession of an honest prayer, the unexpected gift of being seen and known, even amidst our contradictions.

Hope asks something of us: eyes to see what God is doing beneath the surface, ears to hear the whisper we're prone to miss, and patience to stay with the slow work of becoming. Hope does not bypass reality; it illuminates it.

If you're willing to walk through the long path of character formation, hope will find you, too, my friend. So let's begin walking that path together. Here and in the chapters to come I'll leave you with a blessing—an intentionally right-brained, poetic invitation to balance my left-brained analysis. May this blessing be a gesture toward grace; something to be received rather than achieved.

And so, dear friends,

May you read these pages
with open eyes and an honest heart,
curious not just about who you've been,
but who you're becoming.

May the pain you've carried
find a witness
tender enough to hold it
and courageous enough to name it.

May the fractures you've observed in others
not harden your soul with cynicism
but awaken a longing for a life forged in truth—
honest, bold, and tenderhearted.

May your own contradictions
held in secret within you
become invitations,
not to shame, but to grace.

May you abide,
growing in trust,
gazing toward hope,
grounded in love.

May you mature,
shaped slowly and deeply
by the one who carves character
in hidden places.

And may you trust that
even here,
even now,
you are already being transformed.

RESOURCES

At the end of each chapter, recommended books are offered as trusted wells of wisdom from which you can draw even deeper resources for your ongoing journey.

- Steven Garber, *The Fabric of Faithfulness: Weaving Together Belief and Behavior*
- Diane Langberg, *Redeeming Power: Understanding Authority and Abuse in the Church*
- Soong-Chan Rah, *Prophetic Lament: A Call for Justice in Troubled Times*
- Phyllis Tickle, *The Great Emergence: How Christianity Is Changing and Why*

REFLECTION

Throughout the book, these reflections are offered as something you can do on your own, with a friend, or within a small circle of trusted companions.

1. Where has trust been shaken or shattered for you? What causes you real concern in this current moment of reckoning? How has this betrayal of trust impacted you personally? What questions has your own shattered trust left you with?
2. As you consider the relative health or unhealth of the systems you live in, how would you name the problem(s)? How are these impacting you right now? What assumptions, beliefs, or priorities might need to change to allow healing?
3. As you reflect on the meaning of character, what words or themes resonate? Where have you seen character shaped in ways you are grateful for, whether your own or in someone else? Where have

you seen shortcuts or even an absence of character affect your life or the lives of others?

4. How would you describe Christlike character? What do you look for as evidence of strong character?

PRACTICE

Cultivating Acknowledgment, Grief, and Longing for the Sake of Character Change

Throughout the book, the practices at the end of each chapter will build upon one another, at times with some overlap and expansion so you can experience a growing healing and wholeness.

Craft a "Personal Reckoning" Narrative

Take some time to bring to mind a moment of disillusionment or betrayal by another; a moment of inner disappointment at not living up to a standard you'd set for yourself; or perhaps a growing ache amidst the larger, systemic reckoning we're facing.

1. What happened? (This could be quite personal or reflective of a larger cultural movement.)
2. How has this shaped you in both soul and body, in thoughts and feelings, in the ways in which you behave and in your relationships?
3. What has been the cost to you?
4. How do you feel you've moved through it, or how do you continue to feel stuck amidst it?
5. How would you describe the ways you'd like to grow in Christlike character?

Write a Lament

Lament is the biblical response to personal or collective pain. Laments are honest pleas before God, inviting us to name our ache as an antidote to our less-helpful strategies of bypassing, numbing, reacting, or avoiding. Scripture models this in the everyday cries of ordinary human beings like you and me. There are psalms of individual lament—Psalm 3, 5–7, 13, 17, 22, 25–28, 32, 38–39, 42–43, 51, 54–57, 59, 61, 63–64, 69–71, 86, 88, 102, 109, 120, 130, and 140–143. There are also psalms of communal lament—44, 74, 79–80, 83, and 89.[4] What we know is that amidst personal and collective reckonings, we must allow the emotion to move through us in meaningful ways. Lament facilitates this. It invites us to express our grief honestly and unapologetically.

STEP 1: REVIEW SCRIPTURE LAMENTS WITH YOUR EXPERIENCES IN MIND

Read through some of the suggested laments above and see if you might reframe some of your own experiences, emotions, and words in their ancient forms.

STEP 2: COMPOSE A LAMENT

Write your own lament, specifically attending to details of what has affected you.

Describe Your Longing

Laments were often accompanied by longings for justice, safety, accountability, hope, renewed strength, even for peace (what Scripture calls *shalom*). A deep longing of mine is that, despite what we've been through, we'll become—in time—the kind of people described by Jesus in the beatitudes (Matthew 5:1-12) or by Paul in the fruit of the Spirit (Galatians 5:22-23).

1. As you reflect on the themes of character in both these Scripture passages, what do you long for personally?

2. What do you hope for more broadly—for your family, for the church, for the culture as a whole? Write about your longings, and write specifically, allowing your heart to be moved by what emerges.
3. Despite what has happened to you, you can reshape and reauthor your life for the sake of integrity and wholeness. Honestly assess your desire to change at a foundational level. Are you coming to this work with curiosity or resistance? Humble expectancy or anxious urgency? Either way, it's all right—your honesty is what matters.

Be open to what the next chapters might reveal, not merely about other people, but about your own journey of character formation.

PART 1

the foundation of character

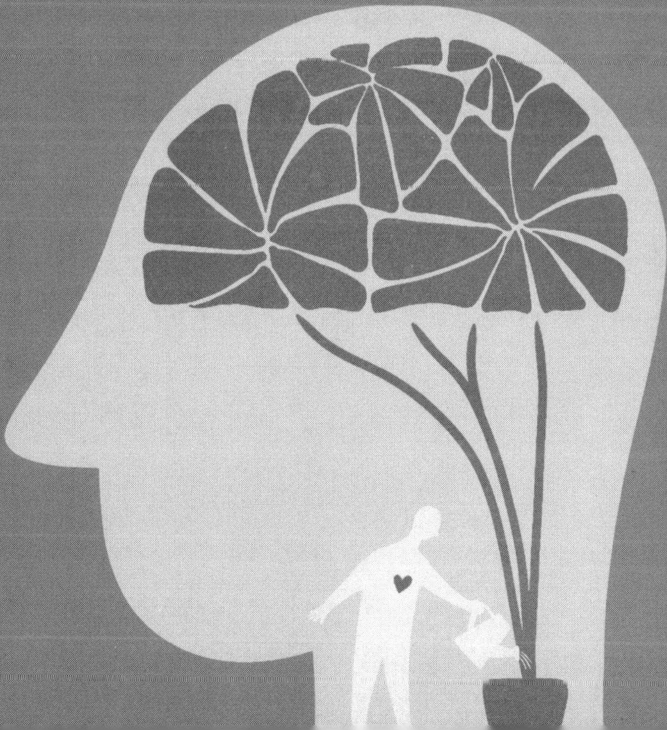

Authentic character change
never announces itself with fanfare.

Rather, it moves like water over stone—
slow, steady, almost imperceptible,
until one day you realize
the landscape of your soul has shifted.

We'd like change to be swift,
like a dam breaking,
sending a rush of water
that carves a new path in an instant.

But more often, it commences slowly,
and with a hush,
in quiet decisions
faithfully made,
over and over again.

It can be frustrating,
this slow work of becoming.
Yet beneath the surface,
where we cannot always see,
the work is being done.
Character does change—
not in an instant,
but in the persistence
of grace and time.

CHAPTER 1

regulated

Building Character Through Connection (Not Perfection)

To be human is to have a heart. You can't not love. So the question isn't whether *you will love something as ultimate; the question is* what *you will love as ultimate. And you are what you love.*

JAMES K. A. SMITH, *YOU ARE WHAT YOU LOVE*

My heart is glad and my tongue rejoices;
my body also will rest secure. . . .
You make known to me the path of life;
you will fill me with joy in your presence.

PSALM 16:9, 11

Sydney had worked for a nonprofit for years, and whenever someone asked her how she liked her job, she'd shrug and say, "Knowing that we're helping people is really gratifying." She never mentioned the pit that formed in her stomach when she heard Jeff, her boss, approach her desk or raise his voice in their weekly staff meetings.

One day over coffee with her friend Anna, Sydney spoke of her spiraling health and panic attacks, prompting Anna to get curious about her satisfaction at work. After Sydney mentioned how Jeff had loudly berated her that morning for letting a typo get through in the annual report, she watched Anna's eyes grow large and her mouth fall open.

"It's fine," Sydney said. "I mean, I don't love being constantly dismissed and disparaged by my boss, but maybe I could be better at my job."

Still Anna's look of astonishment awakened Syndey, validating her pain. "I think your body's telling you something, Syd," Anna said.

Sydney knew it in her gut—*Jeff's bullying isn't right*—but she'd been ignoring the blinking lights on her emotional and somatic dashboard within. She'd been dismissing the disparities in her boss's behavior as one-off mistakes, muting a gut-level urge to take them seriously. After all, she needed the job, and Jeff was an old family friend.

On the surface, Sydney's boss seemed like a good guy—a church elder, a family man, a quick wit. He donated to charity, the team he coached won the Best Sportsmanship Award, and he taught a class on sanctification at his church.

But in her ten years with the company, Sydney had seen Jeff silencing dissent, demanding allegiance, enacting retribution on the disloyal, evading accountability, gaslighting, and more. Within a few weeks of her coffee date with Anna, the nonprofit's board launched an inquiry into Jeff's behavior after receiving multiple complaints from Sydney's coworkers and the organization's clients. The investigating team found that Jeff's aggressive behaviors were something more sinister: patterns of bullying and misbehavior. Dozens of emails and texts further amplified his tendencies toward anger, deceit, and cruelty. And Jeff's closest deputies had become unwitting accomplices, much to their shame.

Upon reading the results of the internal inquiry, Jeff exploded with fury. "That's not who I am!" he exclaimed. (That's the cry of someone whose behavior feels completely reasonable from the inside—what psychologists call *ego-syntonic*: when our patterns fit so comfortably with our self-image that we cannot recognize them as a problem.)

But Jeff was wrong; his character was revealed in habits that had become second nature, habits that he would awaken to only through the eventual shattering of his ego.

Patterns That Reveal Who You Are

Consider this: *Who you are* shows up right here and now—in patterns of thinking, believing, feeling, working, and relating that reveal the deeper and more subtle habits of your heart.

Sure, we're all prone to occasional mistakes and misjudgments. Even people of high character will sometimes disappoint themselves and others. It's inevitable. I recall a friend losing his temper during an important gathering. We knew him to be an even-keeled, non-anxious presence, so the small eruption surprised us all. I grabbed him after the meeting and checked in.

He was embarrassed. Sitting across from me, he was hunched, his face in his hands. "My daughter was hospitalized this weekend for an eating disorder," he said. "I don't know what we're going to do."

Heaving sobs followed, his tears revealing a dad's tender heart and the shame of showing up in a way that violated his deepest sense of propriety. His authentic humility revealed the integrity of his character.

Yes, we're all prone to acting out of stress. Yet when we reflect on Jeff and Sydney, we see a key difference: Jeff's behavior was not a one-time mistake but a recognizable pattern. Calvin University philosopher James K. A. Smith notes that character is "the web of dispositions you've acquired (virtues and vices) that work as automaticities, disposing you to act in certain ways."[1] That's a mouthful, to be sure. But what he's saying is crucial. When it comes to character, we shouldn't just pay attention to one-off behaviors; instead, we should focus on what has become second nature, revealed in the everyday habits and patterns of our lives.

And those habits didn't begin yesterday.

To take character seriously, we need to look deeper and start much earlier.

Because who you are didn't happen overnight. The architecture of your character has been shaped over a lifetime. Who you are is revealed not just in the habits of the heart, but in the hub of what Smith calls the "automaticities"—the workings of the central nervous system.

That's not a recent discovery.

Well before modern advancements in neuroscience and physiology, ancient pastoral psychologists were mapping the inner landscape—and what they discovered has much in common with what we know today about our bodies and brains.

Writing on the lived theology of the desert fathers and mothers of the third and fourth centuries, former archbishop of Canterbury Rowan Williams notes that these cartographers of the soul were not just interested in the outward sinful behavior but in the internal dynamics motivating sin—what they called the "passions." Williams says that they named a "whole realm of instinct, reaction, [and] coping mechanisms" that drive our outward behaviors.[2] In other words, they sensed that the story of our habits is inextricably tied to a churning anxiety within—evidence of self-protection and survival, not safety and security.

If you want to understand character and why people are the way they are, you've got to understand what's happening at this subterranean level within the human heart. You need to pay attention to that realm of instinct, reaction, and coping mechanisms that often operates beneath conscious awareness. Or in more contemporary parlance, you need to pay attention to emotional regulation and dysregulation.

And these states are anchored in your story.

Consider this: Before you had words, your body was already asking, *Am I safe? Am I seen? Am I loved?*

Often, your present character is a direct result of the answer your body was given in those early days, inextricably shaped by these deep, embodied learnings.

If your parents or caregivers consistently responded to your needs, you likely internalized a felt sense of security, allowing you to rest in connection, to explore and take risks as you grew. Through the reliable presence and secure love of your parents or caregivers, you experienced the soothing co-regulation your young and fragile nervous system needed. Think of co-regulation as *connected* regulation—the beautiful grounding and soothing that happens when you're in the presence of another who sees you and deeply cares.

This safe connection may have led to habits of regulation, prompting healthy patterns of reflection, compassion, kindness, patience, long-suffering, even self-awareness—echoes of Christlike character. In other words, this connected regulation manifests in coherence—a life in which your inner world and outer actions sing in harmony.

Consider the beauty of it. This connection orientation means that, from your earliest days, you perceived the world not as a dangerous place that required inner division so you could survive, but as a hospitable place where you felt safe enough to be seen and known, where love could be received and given. This offered you the possibility not just to become a healthy adult but also to become the kind of person who is wholeheartedly devoted in your relationships, vocation, and more.

Conversely, the prolonged absence of co-regulation—either through neglect or abuse—shapes the soul and body much differently. If your early needs were met with inconsistency, criticism, or absence, your body likely learned to adapt. You may have become hypervigilant and people-pleasing, performing for approval, or withdrawing to protect yourself. These early ruptures in care likely led to dysregulation, prompting patterns of reactivity, anxiety, defensiveness, appeasement, grasping after love, even acting out for attention. These are all signs of a character shaped for self-protection and survival, leading to internal division. We see examples all around us. A leader's defensiveness, a parent's relentless overachievement, a therapist's fusion with a client—each can be traced back to those early patterns of division, disconnection, and self-protection.

Such adaptations don't just disappear either; they become the soil out of which habits grow. As these early self-protective strategies endure into adulthood, they become second nature. And the capacity to love becomes *disordered*—which, from a classic theological lens, simply means that our loves are out of order. In other words, instead of learning that love is anchored in connection, we find that love is based on survival and self-protection. This impacts our capacity to love with wholehearted devotion.

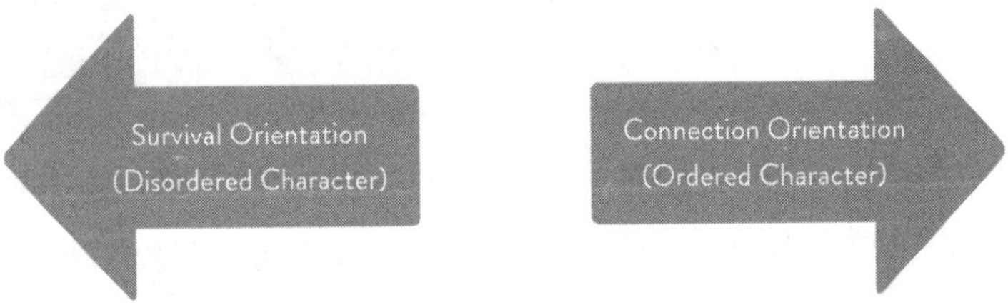

Six Self-Protective Patterns

When our lives are shaped more by survival than connection and when our hearts become divided and disordered, patterns of autonomic nervous system dysregulation are inevitable. This isn't something to beat ourselves up about, but it is an invitation to curiosity because our reflexive responses do have an impact—on us and others.

At times, our patterns will be charged with the self-protective energy of what I call *Storm*, reflecting the activation of our sympathetic nervous system. Here, we might see the instinctive and involuntary response of fight, flight, fawn, and find. At other times, our patterns will reflect the parasympathetic pull to preserve energy or shut down in what I call *Fog*—with its responses of freeze and fold. Fragmented within, these responses reveal how we reflexively and unconsciously navigate a threatening world.

Although it's likely that more could be included, these six core protective patterns reveal what is happening within, beneath the surface, where character is shaped.

Storm (Activation)

In *fight*, we armor up, our bodies postured not just to defend but to attack when necessary. This stance shows up in patterns of irritability, control, defensiveness, argumentativeness, blame-shifting, moral superiority, rigidity, impatience, intimidation, certainty, a desire to win at all costs, and the use of power, words, or righteousness to stay protected. As autonomically charged patterns, they're not easily malleable. So someone might say to a spouse in fight mode, "Stop being so pushy and impatient." But pushiness and impatience have likely worked as a protective shield for that person, perhaps for decades.

This doesn't make the painful impact of it acceptable, but it helps us understand where such behavior comes from.

In *flight*, our patterns look like procrastination, conflict avoidance, distraction, addiction, and spiritual bypassing, yes—but also overplanning, constant busyness, overfunctioning, perfectionism, and compulsive productivity. When people come to me hoping to be less perfectionistic, it'd be easy to offer a cliché like, "Just give yourself more grace" or "You're doing great—you can relax." But a bit of curiosity might reveal that this pattern has operated far longer than they knew, as an early adaptive style to remain safe and secure.

Most people are familiar with fight-or-flight, but there are other everyday patterns that are less often named. In *fawn*, there is an instinctual tendency to lose ourselves in tending to others, but not in a sanctified "self-giving love" sort of way. We may be prone to patterns of people-pleasing, appeasement, excessive agreeableness, self-silencing, overempathy, conflict avoidance, boundary-less caregiving, and anticipatory compliance. While these behaviors may earn us awards in elementary school and leadership positions in adulthood, they may also reflect a nervous system stuck in an early developmental pattern of pleasing a parent who is anxious, angry, or neglectful.

Find is yet another autonomic, reflexive response, an instinctual pattern of emotional enmeshment and dependency, seen in excessive neediness, clinginess, reassurance seeking, fear of abandonment, collapsing boundaries, overdisclosure, dependency on approval, emotional fusion, and confusing proximity with safety. And while we might want to tell someone stuck in this pattern, "Stop being so needy," it's not that easy. This, too, is indexed into a person's overall style of self-protection, and it's not easily shifted.

Fight, flight, fawn, and find implicate the sympathetic nervous system, your body in active self-protection. This is a state I call Storm because you're internally hyperaroused.[3] And because these states are physiological, instinctual, and unconscious, they're often ego-syntonic. As we saw with Jeff, that means you might not even notice the pervasive impact these states have on your everyday ways of living and relating. *This is just who I am, who I've always been*, you reason.

Even though Jeff thought of himself as a good guy, a committed Christian, and a generally self-aware leader, he needed to reckon with an internal drive to fight which had long been his most basic instinct. This was revealed not just in his harrowing work habits but later in abusive patterns within his marriage and workplace.

Tragically, Jeff's sense of self-awareness was largely superficial; he mistook the "fight" mask he'd worn for so long as his true self. Dysregulation and inner disorder had become "normal," and he was unaware that his reflexive patterns of intimidation, moral superiority, and need for control drove so many of his interactions. Friends even colluded with his sense of self, affirming him as a "strong leader" who was frequently misunderstood by people with "daddy issues." This is why, for Jeff and so many others, a surface-level self-awareness doesn't equate to self-regulation.

"I can't believe I've been stuck in *fight* my whole life," Jeff would say much later, a bit stunned to consider its abiding role in his life. "It became the only reality I knew."

Jeff's capacity for repentance would grow as he recognized the truth. He wasn't merely a leader who had a bad day now and then—he was governed by forces within that had been established long before, to keep him safe as he grew up amidst fatherlessness and chaos. He was animated by a fight instinct that was born out of a tough home life and an early vow to make it despite the odds. This led to relational patterns with dire moral consequences.

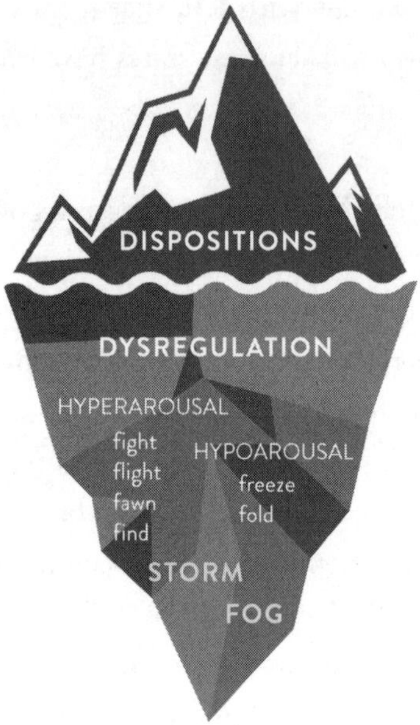

Fog (Shutdown)

And deeper still within this subterranean layer of the psyche are patterns of *freeze* and *fold*. *Freeze* is sometimes described as a deer-in-the-headlights sensation—an instinctual and involuntary immobility. It might be experienced as numbness, indecision, withdrawal, passivity, invisibility, learned helplessness, low affect, and the quiet belief that it's safer not to move at all. As Sydney reflected on her experience working with Jeff at the nonprofit, she realized how even though she knew it in her gut—*it isn't right*—she'd ignored her own intuition. She froze in order to survive. Eventually she would see that her particular default patterns, including the freeze instinct, were learned under the cruel thumb of an abusive father. Her own character—often described as modest and kind but better named as muted and deferential—was fueled by self-protection rather than other-centered love. This led to what is sometimes called a chronic, functional freeze, a state in which a person remains outwardly capable and productive while inwardly numb, constrained, and disconnected from felt vitality. For Sydney, becoming aware of this would lead to her own humility and growth.

Finally, when the situation is dire, our body sometimes responds by *folding*, the quiet closing of the self when staying open no longer feels survivable. It's not laziness or apathy. It's the body's way of saying, "It's too much!" *Fold* is experienced as low energy, heaviness, depression, withdrawal, fatigue, diminished curiosity, and a wish to simply disappear as a means of surviving. And with this pattern, too, there are no clichés or quick fixes that can undo what's been functionally normal for a long time.

These six patterns—fight, flight, fawn, find, freeze, and fold—often shift from short-term survival responses to chronic and long-term ways of navigating a fraught world, the proverbial mask becoming the only face we know. And once these autonomic responses become second nature, they're hard to see, as both Jeff and Sydney discovered. We may even baptize them as righteous. Some of the typical go-to places for self-awareness—the Enneagram, the Myers-Briggs assessment, StrengthsFinder, 360 reviews, or standard leadership or church planting assessments—won't reveal these subterranean dynamics. We may even exhaust ourselves trying to fix our anger, perfectionism, procrastination, or perceived laziness, using tools, techniques, and practices that don't address these inner patterns and don't recognize their core adaptive function within the evolving story of our nervous systems. This is a recipe for exasperation, and I see so many people here, feeling stuck without a solution.

But there is hope, my friends. Our nervous system is not set in stone; our learned automaticities can change with curiosity and compassion. Over time, it's possible to reorient ourselves away from disconnection and back toward connection, creating the conditions for the character change we long for.

Devotion and Disorder

Character, you see, is not ultimately behavioral. It's relational. In some ways, then, Christlike character, too, is more *caught* than *taught*.

Of course, a mix of factors contribute to Christlike character and wholehearted devotion: worship, discipleship, prayer, community, catechesis, and more. I'm not at all suggesting moral formation and wise instruction are replaceable. But these are actually built on a foundation of connection—and wither when it is absent.

Jesus said, "Anyone who listens to my teaching and follows it is wise, like a person who builds a house on solid rock. Though the rain comes in torrents and the floodwaters rise and the winds beat against that house, it won't collapse because it is built on bedrock" (Matthew 7:24-25, NLT). A safe and secure foundation doesn't immunize us to every storm that might hit or do damage, but it fortifies us.

I know what you're likely thinking: *Don't tell me my lack of perfection is the cause of my child's struggles, Chuck! No parent is perfect!* Indeed. I've got a long list of parenting foibles. But this isn't about perfection; it's about connection. We don't have to get it right every time.[4]

The key is this: When we don't get it right, we get to circle back around and reconnect. We get to check in and re-tune. Perfection doesn't build the secure foundation. Connection does, even when we mess up. A woman I was seeing for counseling told me, "My father was anxious and angry at times, but I could always count on him to come back around and ask me about it." She experienced ruptures in connection, but her secure foundation was built on repair and reconnection. That phrase—"I could always count on him"—makes all the difference.

We can't minimize the painful reality, however, of a life built on an insecure foundation. What happens to infants who can't count on their parents to reconnect? The unreliable presence and insecure love of their parents or caregivers mean that co-regulation isn't available, prompting babies to self-soothe. To be sure, every baby comforts themselves to some degree, but imagine for a moment infants who have no one reliable to turn to, to be seen or held by. It's scary for little ones—even if they aren't conscious of it. These children do not learn coherence but contradiction, dividing the self—one part performing for connection, the other burying what feels too vulnerable to be seen. Their survival styles will likely be reflected in a single pattern or a mix of the six patterns of fight, flight, fawn, find, freeze, or fold.

But what if these patterns become so ingrained that they take over, dominating the entire personality? Interestingly, psychologists call deeply ingrained patterns personality disorders, noting that they are characterological, which means that they've come to define one's character. They represent such a heightened state of inner division that things have gotten "out of order" within, becoming disruptive not just internally but relationally as well.

It's critical to see that personality disorders are not character defects but ingrained patterns emerging over time, shaped by an interplay of biology and lived experience. Our biology provides the construction material, our childhood environment builds from there, and our resulting sense of safety (or lack thereof) determines which behaviors we rely on and which we deem unsafe. This is why a secure foundation is so vital.[5] Personality disorders are not labels that we haphazardly apply—they're extreme manifestations of survival patterns. And while these lived patterns can be harmful to ourselves or others, requiring accountability, understanding them can lead to empathy.

I've been working with people exhibiting personality disorders for more than twenty-five years, and a subset seems to show up more frequently in churches, organizations, and leadership assessments. Looking through a trauma-informed, empathetic lens, here are some of the disorders I frequently see:

Borderline personality disorder—protection through intensity. If love has been unpredictable—offered, then withdrawn—desperation takes root. Emotional extremes become both a protest against abandonment and a test of devotion, forcing connection while ensuring no one can get close enough to inflict final betrayal.

Histrionic personality disorder—protection through performance. When worth seems contingent on attention, life becomes a stage. Exaggeration and charm secure a place in the spotlight, and being noticed substitutes for being truly known.

Narcissistic personality disorder—protection through grandiosity. If early wounds suggest one is insignificant, a larger-than-life persona forms as armor. The pursuit of attention, admiration, and achievement drowns out the quiet terror of shame and unworthiness, securing love on external terms.

Avoidant personality disorder—protection through retreat. If rejection has cut too deep, avoidance becomes a shelter. By withdrawing from the possibility of failure, shame, or disappointment, the individual ensures that pain is kept at bay, even at the cost of connection.

Dependent personality disorder—protection through submission. When autonomy feels dangerous or overwhelming, dependence on another becomes the answer. By yielding, pleasing, and clinging, the individual ensures they are never left to navigate life alone.

Obsessive-compulsive personality disorder (OCPD)—protection through control. In a world that feels chaotic or unreliable, order becomes salvation. Perfectionism, rigidity, and an unwavering need for structure provide the illusion of mastery, ensuring that unpredictability—and the fear it brings—is minimized.

Recognizing how hearts created for wholehearted devotion can shift toward division, disconnection, and disorder is critical for our understanding of deep character change. This spectrum includes all of us, and studying it provides a growing sense of clarity around the subterranean dynamics of the human heart.[6]

While personality disorders do not equate to character defects, we can't ignore the importance of personal accountability. Living a disordered life hurts. It hurts the people suffering from it, and it hurts and sometimes harms those in their orbit.

Empathy and Accountability

Maybe you've been hurt by someone who has one or more of these disordered styles of relating. I'm not at all endeavoring to condone the harm these issues cause. In fact, if you are in a relationship that is coercive, controlling, or abusive, your priority is not that person's character change. Your priority is your own protection. So by all means, with the help of a friend, pastor, or mental health practitioner, get whatever you need to be safe.

We are each responsible for our own actions, so while our hearts stretch toward empathy as we understand the roots of relational patterns, we're also mindful of their profound impact. Jeff was elevated on the narcissistic spectrum. His unexamined survival strategies, fused with institutional and spiritual power, led to behaviors that were rightly named as abusive, requiring accountability. And while it would be easy to label Jeff's actions merely as coping techniques, they were also rightly named as sin.

When we name the dynamics of the heart through the lens of our brains and bodies, some people might bristle and say, "You are soft on sin." I've personally heard that. However, what I've noticed is that, among those who claim to take sin seriously, there is a serious lack of curiosity and clarity around what fuels our besetting habits.

Some tend to settle for what Dallas Willard calls "sin management"—a surface-level game of soul Whac-A-Mole that represents a shallow attempt at assuaging the anxious undercurrent fueling habits and behavior.[7] This shallow sin-management approach often leads to cheap grace in the form of quick fixes.

On paper, Jeff had a robust theology of sin. In practice, he hoped a brief sabbatical and a contrite-sounding general apology to his staff might pave the way for a quick comeback. In my experience, I've seen the most resistance to change from those most committed to strong theological formulations of sin. Ironically, those most fluent in the language of sin are often least prepared for the loss of control that real transformation requires. The body knows what the theology resists: Deep change threatens identity, reputation, and power. Here, primal patterns of self-protection kick in. Sadly, repentance is often compressed into statements and sabbaticals while the underlying patterns remain untouched.

Sin is not merely a behavioral violation, as some assume, but our habitual participation in patterns of self-protection and disconnection—from self, others, and God. While we might empathize as we discover the insecure roots of disordered patterns, we can't minimize the hurt and harm they cause: addictions, abuse, betrayal, bullying, and much more.

But here's the challenge—when disordered patterns are named, the nervous system often engages the old survival responses. In Jeff's case, this led him to armor up. Deflect. Avoid. Blame. If this reminds you of someone you know, you're likely aware that this internal dynamic shuts down any possibility of transformative change, rendering most early apologies or efforts merely performative, ego-preserving, and image-managing. If you're reading this as someone who is hoping for deep change yourself, I invite you to recognize these dynamics in your own heart, not as a source of shame but as a gateway to hope.

Deep character change requires a person to step completely away from anything that seeks to preserve their ego-syntonic self-image. This might mean leaving a leadership role, not merely for weeks or months, but for much longer—long enough to reestablish regulation, safety, security, and connection, the conditions in which honest words, real repentance, and genuine change can flow. Even the apostle Paul—the chief architect of a theology of grace—needed three years in the desert for grace to deal with the depths of his pharisaic formation. Quick comebacks circumvent deeper dynamics of the heart, compromising the possibility of real transformation.

This is hard but ultimately hopeful, especially for those committed to enduring transformation.

Transformed Through Love

"You are what you love," James K. A. Smith writes.[8] And while Smith wasn't referring to the human nervous system, his insight into the habits of the heart is spot-on. Our capacity to love, and love well, requires a secure foundation. Absent it, we can't love fully, and we might even harm others.

That's a hard reality to swallow. It was for me. It's understandable if, at this point, you feel like you're doomed to disordered living because of a painful past. But I hope instead it invites curiosity and compassion for yourself, even for the fraught, early formative moments you may have experienced. Consider this hopeful perspective: Understanding how your loves were shaped and your habits were formed is key to transformative character change. You are not doomed by your painful past, and there is no expiration date on the possibility of repair and reconnection.

For decades, I've worked with people who've exhausted themselves with New Year's resolutions and novel practices, strict Bible-reading regimens and high-commitment small group studies, devout devotional habits and disciplined lives. But many are left with inevitable questions: *Why am I not changing? Why do I still have such a temper? Why do I react so strongly? Why do I procrastinate so much? Why am I so obsessive?* I get the effort, but effort alone built on a foundation of insecurity and anxiety leads to futility.

Like many of us, Jeff spent years in what he thought were noble efforts at becoming a stronger leader and a better person—engaging in Scripture reading and men's gatherings, even participating in Enneagram staff retreats and personal journaling—all prior to his crisis. Yet it was his unaddressed dysregulation that fueled his rapid-fire, self-resourcing program, blinding him to the deeper forces that drove his behavior.

In addition to stepping away from his leadership role, Jeff began meeting regularly with Bill, who had retired several years before from the CEO position Jeff now held. A wise and seasoned leader, Bill became a safe person with whom Jeff could process the findings of the internal report and examine the anxious drive that compelled Jeff to be so hard on others. This was a critical part of his restoration.

Why is walking alongside a safe and wise person so critical as you seek to develop your character? Your body is designed to naturally relax its protective mechanisms in the presence of someone you can trust. When another person offers a calm, steady, nonjudgmental presence, your defenses soften, allowing you to access the parts of yourself you normally hide or protect. In this co-regulating space, character change can finally take root in a body and soul that feels safe enough to be honest, vulnerable, and receptive to grace.

Once Bill finally helped Jeff realize that he had been bringing his fight strategy to the change process, Jeff relinquished, worn out and embarrassed. That's when he finally surrendered his futile and exhausting efforts, instead daring to be known—engaging in the vulnerable relational work that would once and for all begin to reorder and reconcile his inner divisions. In time, Jeff found the courage to get curious about this fight strategy—humbled that it had been a resource to protect himself in his earliest years, and heartbroken that it had become a harmful way of relating to others into adulthood.

The Scottish preacher and theologian Thomas Chalmers (1780–1847) talked about the "expulsive power of a new affection," the idea that the best way to break free from something that has a grasp on your heart isn't to try harder to push it away but to let your heart be captured by a stronger, better love that slowly makes the old one lose its grip.[9] But this requires courageous vulnerability—a heart open to love, care, and delight.

In harmony with Chalmers, Rowan Williams notes that early church sages didn't remedy defensiveness and reactivity with quick fixes but with sturdy love, a "mutual gaze of love and delight: the flow and return and overflow of divine life."[10] These early Christians weren't interested in putting Band-Aids on sin—they believed that the cure for extreme anxiety and insecurity of the soul was a deeper security in God.

Here again we see that character change isn't taught but caught—in the context of vulnerable love and honest relationship. Only a new and deeper source of love can help us break free. My hope is that you, too, can break free from the grip of old affections as your heart awakens to a pathway beyond fight and flight, please and appease, stuck and shutdown. I know no other path than this slow and vulnerable one.

I've sat with folks whose disordered patterns caused disruptions personally and relationally, and whose self-protective strategies took time to relax. Can you find the courage to stay with the questions, the reckoning, the storms within, rather than seeking a quick work-around? Can you find your way to a healing relationship where shame will dissolve and secure love will grow?

Grace isn't a race to the finish line. You can't force character change. Reckonings and reformations—personal and collective—take time. A sacred repatterning within needs to happen, and it can with your consent. If you long to change—or long to see someone you love change—it begins here, at this foundational level, as you find your way into the safe arms of divine Love, as you are held by others who want what's best for you, as your loves are reordered at the depths.

Love will help you find your way Home.

And so, dear friends,

May you find the courage to stay.
To stay with the ache, the questions, the reckoning.
To resist the quick comeback and embrace the long return.

May you find the courage to name the storms within without shame
and befriend the fog rather than flee from it.

May you honor the slow healing of your nervous system
and the sacred repatterning of love.

May you trust the wisdom of your longing,
the longing for coherence more than the charade,
for connection more than control.

And may you know the secure Love
that fosters lasting regulation,
nurtures honest relationships,
and grows deep roots.

RESOURCES

- Aimie Apigian, *The Biology of Trauma: How the Body Holds Fear, Pain, and Overwhelm, and How to Heal It*
- James F. Masterson, *The Search for the Real Self: Unmasking the Personality Disorders of Our Age*
- James K. A. Smith, *You Are What You Love: The Spiritual Power of Habit*

REFLECTION

1. What are you sensing about the ways character change differs from growth in emotional health, boundaries, or spiritual practices?
2. How does Sydney's response to Jeff's managerial style—shut-down, avoidance, and silent discomfort—illustrate why it's so important to examine one's own character? Why do you think we tend to miss or ignore these dynamics?
3. What are some rationalizations or minimizations you've heard that dismiss real faults or flaws of character?

4. As you consider your own early story of regulation (or dysregulation), how do you think your body's felt sense of safety shaped your habits over time? How does understanding the source and shape of people's habits, even from their earliest moments, impact the way you understand their character and the change process?
5. Like so many people, Jeff thought he was engaging in good practices, even ones designed to make him more self-aware. However, he did not realize that he was living in fight mode and hadn't yet taken the time to get curious about the origins of this internalized, reflexive response. Which of the six F's—fight, flight, fawn, find, freeze, and fold—do you most relate to? How has your spiritual journey become entangled with this autonomic pattern?
6. Renewed safety and connection create the conditions for a regulated nervous system, which leads to growing habits of Christlike character formation. These are core realities (not mere strategies to tame sin or manage behavior). As you consider how safety and connection can change us from the inside out, do you have a story of how you've seen real, lasting change in you or someone else? How does this process expand your vision for real character change—for yourself and for others?

PRACTICE

Cultivating Safety for the Sake of Character Change

Tracking

This brief practice helps you notice your nervous system in real time—whether you're in Storm (activation) or Fog (shutdown)—by tracking subtle bodily cues and protective patterns you may not yet be conscious of. It's not merely about calming but about cultivating awareness and compassion as the first step toward regulation and change.

STEP 1: NOTICE YOUR BODY

Ask yourself, *What do I notice in my body right now?* (It might be tightness, pressure, urgency, aggression, withdrawing, heaviness, numbness, etc.)

No need to interpret. Just track your internal energy.

STEP 2: NOTICE ENERGY AND DIRECTION

Now notice the direction of your energy:

Does it feel like energy is rising, pushing, bracing, or mobilizing?

Or does it feel like energy is dropping, fading, slowing, or shutting down?

This shift in energy is often easier to sense than emotion.

STEP 3: ATTEMPT TO NAME THE PATTERN

If the energy feels activated or urgent, you may be in Storm.

See if any of these feel familiar right now:

Fight—irritation, defensiveness, inner arguing

Flight—restlessness, distraction, urgency to escape

Fawn—appeasing, over-agreeing, managing others

Find—searching, clamoring, soliciting

If the energy feels heavy, distant, or collapsed, you may be in Fog:

Freeze—stuck, blank, unable to decide or move

Fold—withdrawn, hopeless, resigned, quietly overwhelmed

You're not diagnosing—just noticing what fits.

STEP 4: ADD A SENTENCE OF KINDNESS

Before doing anything else, try one of these simple phrases:

"Something in me is trying to protect me right now."

"Something in me is trying to send a message right now."

"This reaction makes sense, given what I've lived."

Let that land in your body for a breath or two.

STEP 5: STAY CURIOUS (NOT FIXING)

End by asking—not answering—two simple questions:

- What might your nervous system be responding to right now?
- What need might this part of you be communicating—fewer demands, more space, or gentle support?

Then stop. Tracking alone is the practice.

Cultivating a Felt Sense of Safety

Character change starts with what I call the autonomic basics, the body-and-brain-based essentials that create the conditions for this crucial shift from survival to connection. We take for granted these autonomic basics like safety, connection, rest, steadiness, delight, and peace. Cultivating character change begins here, as our survival strategies are relaxed and as we discover the "still waters" and "green pastures" (see Psalm 23:2) of deep autonomic rest.

Too often, we reduce character change to behavioral change—*I'll switch a few things around in my life, and all will be well.* But if your nervous system is in a posture of self-protection or disconnection, nothing you do will stick.

If you're curious about how people change—or if you're reading to engage your own change process—this is as good a place as any to begin. The autonomic basics (which foster that needed inner security) nurture a connection orientation, which becomes the foundation of new habits and practices, and lasting change. This is true whether you're a survivor of trauma, a perpetrator of abuse, or simply someone who has sensed some inner resistance to change despite the many things you've tried.

How do you build this foundation? It begins by returning to the core needs you might have missed so long ago: feeling safe, seen, soothed, and secure.[11] In this exercise, you'll cultivate a felt sense of safety, and you'll return to the other three S's in future chapters.

Safety whispers to your body, *It's okay to change. Your defenses can relax.* You can begin to open yourself to the possibility of newness, connection, and transformation, not least because your body is beginning to find its way to regulation.

STEP 1: SEEK A SAFE PERSON

Character transformation doesn't depend on performance or willpower. Instead, it is rooted in safety, which begins by connecting with safe people—a process called co-regulation. The presence of a calm and nonjudgmental person provides the safety needed to soften your defenses and open yourself to change.

Is there someone (a friend, mentor, spiritual director, therapist, etc.) with whom you might be able to feel safe? How might you take the courageous step, as Sydney did with Anna, to establish a personal or professional relationship with such a person?

STEP 2: SEEK SAFETY THROUGH SELF-REGULATION

Safety can also be fostered through gentle and sustained self-regulation, which creates the internal stability needed to face hard truths without collapsing into shame or reacting from fear. When you can calm your own nervous system, you gain the clarity and courage required for honest reflection, making space for the slow, steady work of character transformation. I invite you to practice communicating safety through the following self-regulation exercise:

- Sit in a comfortable chair with your feet on the floor, placing your nondominant hand on your chest and your dominant hand on your abdomen.

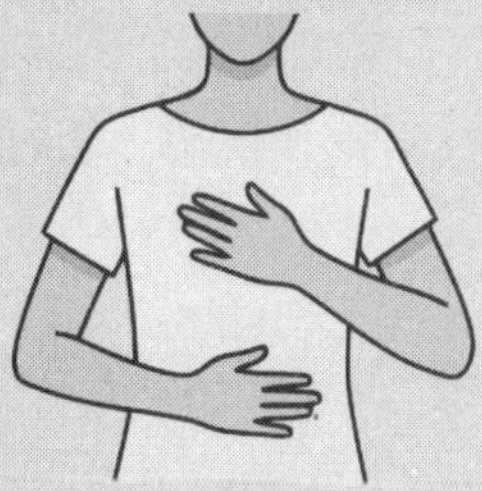

SAFE

- Begin to breathe—inhaling for four seconds (expanding your belly), holding for seven seconds, and exhaling for eight seconds.
- This practice is more powerful when you also have a felt sense of God's presence within and/or around you. If it feels right to you, you might expand your breathing exercise with a foundational practice of seeking to foster felt safety with God, drawing on this passage from Psalm 4:8:

  Lord (inhale for four seconds)

  make me dwell (hold for seven)

  in safety (exhale for eight)

As you sense your body relaxing in either of these practices, you might whisper to yourself, "I'm okay; I'm not in danger. I don't need to control my world. I don't need to fight or flee." You might do this with a safe friend, allowing their gentle presence to confirm this reality for you. Slowly, your posture toward the world can change. This won't happen overnight because your body's self-protection systems didn't activate overnight. Feeling safe will take time, but it will happen.

Many folks I've worked with—particularly men on the narcissistic spectrum—have little idea how regularly their bodies feel threatened. This little exercise may seem silly at first. But if our earliest attachment maps left us feeling threatened, orienting our bodies and brains toward safety is crucial for change.

CHAPTER 2

rooted

Encouraging Authenticity in a World That Performs It

Selves—goes itself; myself *it speaks and spells,*
Crying Whát I dó is me: for that I came.
GERARD MANLEY HOPKINS

I pray that out of his glorious riches he may strengthen you with power through his Spirit in your inner being, so that Christ may dwell in your hearts through faith. And I pray that you, being rooted and established in love, may have power, together with all the Lord's holy people, to grasp how wide and long and high and deep is the love of Christ.
EPHESIANS 3:16-18

Jordan's raw and unvarnished takes on life grew his TikTok and Instagram platforms into the tens of thousands before he turned thirty-five. The son of a popular preacher whose teaching style appealed to an older generation, Jordan used his social media to boil spirituality down to the basics, and he offered it with apparent sincerity—stripped-down truths for a weary, scrolling generation.

Beautiful visuals were behind him whenever he was recording: sun-faded wood decks, ocean backdrops, and softly filtered vulnerability. He'd sit cross-legged in a worn tank top, surfboard propped behind him, gritty beard and vintage hat perfectly disheveled—speaking in gravelly tones about presence, healing, and "unlearning who the world told you to be." In his curated videos, every frame clamored after authenticity—albeit a faux vulnerability that was postured and polished.

Jordan's preacher dad always told him he could be whoever he wanted to be. "Chase your dreams," he'd say, with a voice full of conviction, believing he was doing the right thing. Jordan was grateful—and he took his dad at his word, venturing out, taking risks, reinventing himself again and again, on camera and in life.

But beneath the curated freedom, Jordan nurtured a quiet ache.

His dad, for all his words, was rarely there. Jordan was grateful for his father's cheerleading, but underneath he rarely felt connected to or known by his dad, who preached at eight services over the weekends and was rarely home in the evenings. A quick "Way to go, buddy" wasn't enough to quell a quiet voice within that whispered, *But what if I'm venturing in the wrong direction?* His dad did cheer him on, but he wasn't the present, attuned, wise guide who could accompany his son into inner lands unknown.

So Jordan found the relational mirror he needed in his iPhone camera, and he learned to self-soothe with performance. His dad was a preacher for a prim-and-proper world, and Jordan simply wanted to offer a picture of faith that could be messy and honest. And yet, even his attempt at "honest" faith felt postured and performed, ultimately becoming exhausting. His performative authenticity couldn't soothe the emptiness he'd feel when the camera turned off—when it felt like he disappeared.

What's Real and What's "Fauxnerable"

Performative authenticity isn't exactly new; it has just evolved, offered with a slick combination of finesse and fauxnerability these days.

In my early days as a newly ordained minister and licensed therapist, the suspicion of therapy was palpable, especially in my particular ecclesial orbit. I'd often invite friends and colleagues to be more vulnerable, and they'd look at me as if I were inviting them to undress in public.

But over the years, I sensed a subtle shift. I'd hear from colleagues in ministry that they were beginning to do counseling or reading authors they'd once seen as questionable.

I was heartened.

But in the past decade, I've noticed something different—something unsettling. While consulting more broadly on pastoral health, I often encounter leaders who are fluent in the language of therapy. They talk about their desire to be authentic, vulnerable, and humble, about the virtues and vices of their Enneagram type, even about their own counselors. They might share a seemingly vulnerable part of their story in a public presentation or sermon. And yet I sometimes see and hear about the contradictions: their inability to receive feedback, their relational unavailability and misattunement, even their use of Enneagram typing or therapeutic language to evade personal accountability.

It's a disorienting experience—where there was once resistance, there is now embrace, but often a performative embrace. A performative authenticity. A false vulnerability—what I've come to name *fauxnerability*.

Authenticity is one of those words that is often misused and confused. But fostering real authenticity is core to character change.

What is authenticity? And how might it serve as a crucial building block of character?

True authenticity, at its core, is learning to trust and follow an internal compass, implanted by God, that whispers what's true about your essence. It is not something that needs to be acquired or attained, performed or paraded, but something that unfolds. Our work, then, is to learn how to decode and separate fauxnerability from true authenticity—and to do that, we must be clear on what authenticity is, as well as how we began to lose it and why we began to perform in the first place.

To be authentic is to stay connected to the quiet voice within that knows what is true, even before you can articulate it. Consider, for example, how most parents, without even deciding to, see their children as unique, each one born into the world with their very own imprint of God's image. When parents make room for difference, curiosity, and voice, they help each child become the author of their own unique life, grounded in a self that is both rooted and growing. This is not self-centeredness; it's *soul*-centeredness—a lifelong unfolding of integrity from the inside out.

Trauma and addiction expert Dr. Gabor Maté describes authenticity this way:

> The elemental root of "authenticity" is the Greek *autos*, or "self," closely related to "author" and "authority." To be authentic is to be true to a sense of self arising from one's own unique and genuine essence, to be plugged into this inner GPS and to navigate from it.[1]

Maté names something rooted and essential—an internal navigation system, a homing beacon which leads us back to our true selves. In many ways, Maté's definition alludes to what the nineteenth-century English priest and poet Gerard Manley Hopkins coined as *inscape*; that is, your unmistakable essence, an irreducible uniqueness woven into you by God. It's the *you* you live out of when you're deeply rooted—not pulled by emotional, relational, and performative winds, but grounded in your deepest self.

This idea can be traced back even further. Duns Scotus was a thirteenth-century Franciscan friar, philosopher, and theologian who called this idea *haecceitas*, an old Latin word that translates roughly to "this-ness"—as in, the this-ness of a thing:

This oak tree, singular in its beauty.
This tulip, wholly its own.
This you, unlike any other.

Inscape is the invitation of a lifetime to unearth, inhabit, explore, and cultivate your unique internal geography, your particular inner landscape, not just for yourself but for a flourishing world.[2] "For we are God's handiwork [*poiēma*]," says the apostle Paul, "created in Christ Jesus to do good works, which God prepared in advance for us to do" (Ephesians 2:10). You are Christ's one-of-a-kind poem, your God-breathed life inimitably yours.

That's quite different from the artificial authenticity we see evolving before our eyes, isn't it?

So how did we get here? What went wrong?

Inscape Lost

Jordan's father told him to be himself, but he wasn't present with Jordan to hold the inevitable questions that would arise, or even to guide him into the depths of his unique soul.

Sadly, many of us didn't experience attunement to our budding authenticity from our parents. Instead, we experienced emotional absence, disengagement, or a hands-off posture that felt like freedom but functioned as disconnection. This can shape authenticity in profound ways:

- *Emotional unavailability:* Parents who are emotionally distant, preoccupied, or numb. A child's excitement, fear, or sorrow meets a blank stare or distracted response, prompting the child to conclude their inner world does not matter.
- *Premature independence:* Praising children for being "so mature" or "so self-sufficient" while quietly expecting them to handle emotions, decisions, or struggles alone. They may learn to bypass their need for support and connection, mistaking isolation for strength.
- *Non-intervention in distress:* Failing to step in when a child is overwhelmed, bullied, or confused, assuming they will "figure it out." The child may internalize the message that their struggles are theirs alone to carry.
- *Low attunement to uniqueness:* Offering little curiosity about a child's emerging personality, passions, or questions. Without reflective mirroring, children may struggle to know who they are at all.
- *Conflict avoidance:* Withdrawing rather than engaging when tension arises. Instead of learning repair and differentiation,

children may learn that difficult emotions create distance rather than connection.
- *Neglect masked as autonomy:* Giving children total freedom—and believing this is positive because it isn't controlling—while failing to provide them with the steady presence that allows exploration to feel safe. Authenticity requires both freedom and attuned guidance.

For others of us, our authenticity was stifled, perhaps by controlling or enmeshed parents and caregivers. This can happen in a number of ways:

- *Dismissing emotions:* Saying things like "You're fine" or "Don't be so sensitive." This teaches children to distrust their emotional reality.
- *Conditional affection:* Giving love or approval only when children behave, perform, or comply. ("Good girls don't talk back.") They learn to perform for connection rather than express their unique, God-created self.
- *Overriding instincts:* Forcing children to hug someone they're uncomfortable with, or pushing them to smile when they're sad. This signals that their bodies' cues and boundaries can't be trusted.
- *Parentification or role reversal:* Making children responsible for a parent's emotional well-being. Children may suppress their own needs to maintain the relationship, forgoing authenticity just to maintain connection, albeit an anxious one.
- *Punishing curiosity or creativity:* Responding to children's questions, imagination, or nonconforming behavior with

irritation or ridicule. They may learn that self-expression is unsafe or unwanted.

Many of us live with the feeling of being misunderstood by those who raised us. A financial planner I spoke with told me she was the "oddball" in the family. "No one liked numbers and puzzles like I did," she said, a sullen glaze in her eyes. Now in her forties, she rarely goes home for holidays because of how alone and unseen she feels there. And yet she'll still parade her financial success before her parents to elicit some recognition.

I am not immune. As recently as my fiftieth birthday, I wondered if my aging parents would ever really *get* me. In many ways, I see aspects of each of my parents in me—my dad's dry wit, my mom's helpfulness. But as many who know us would say, I'm entirely different from them. I felt it as a kid. "I don't know where you came from," my mom would say jokingly when I shared with her some vocational aspirations in my early twenties. This was a recurring sentiment as they watched the arc of my career unfold, wondering how *their son* turned out like this. Even though it hurt, I can understand why they parented like they did. They—like so many parents of their generation—weren't apprenticed in nurturing authenticity. Nor did they know to cultivate the uniqueness they saw in me from an early age.

But the fact remained: I longed to be seen not as odd or an outlier within the family, but as a profoundly unique and carefully crafted image bearer of an immensely creative God. Absent a parent who is committed to nurturing our authenticity—our inner GPS—we are left to our own devices: morphing, appeasing, clamoring, and chasing after a version of authenticity that we hope will lead us to the love we so desperately need.

Inscape and the Shape of Your Character

I sat across from Gary in late summer of 1997 wearing the Oxford University sweatshirt I'd purchased just weeks prior while studying there—a performative garment to impress others. I'd wear it on the outside to quell the growing shame on the inside. To become *someone*, I thought, I needed to be an academic, and I needed to display my acumen, on a sweatshirt for all to behold.

In the pastoral care class I had taken under Gary the semester prior, I had sat in the back, barely attentive, cracking jokes about how useless it was. Now, after a summer of attempting to prove myself worthy of PhD work overseas, I sat before Gary as my only hope.

"It's never enough," he said, with a knowing grin. "The grades, the effort, the appearance. . . . It's not working, is it?"

Gary knew. I'm not sure how he knew, except that I suspect he'd tried at one point too.

At twenty-seven, I was lost. The long-held grief of not feeling known spilled over, and he held space for me. Gary created room for my illusions to come crashing down. He may have been the first mentor in my life not to indulge my appetite for more, not to offer the customary clichés I'd become used to—compliments affirming my intellect and gifts, words that only served to propel my chase. Instead, Gary invited me to slow way down, to pause my PhD aspirations and get curious about what fueled my pressurized and performative life.

It was this invitation to honesty that allowed me to give up the life I thought I should live and finally begin listening to the story God was writing within me. Gary didn't know it, but his gentle presence and deep recognition created the early conditions for my own reshaped character.

The preeminent twentieth-century psychologist Carl Jung connected our unlived lives to the underdeveloped or unlived lives of our parents.[3] That's not to place blame, but to inspire curiosity. Jung believed, as I do, that our best chance to become ourselves begins in childhood, with parents whose own wholeness inspires our own. I'd received little guidance from a dad who himself was withering in his vocation and a mom whose delight in her kids couldn't quell the ache of a loveless marriage and her own unprocessed grief.

My parents loved me as best they could. But I also carried an unbearable burden—they hoped a child could save their failing marriage. They were unattuned to my needs and my unique inscape because they were hoping a son might meet their unmet longings. It would take a lot of patience and curiosity to unearth the consequences of this for my life. Here, too, I'd need to get honest—uncomfortably honest—as I began to engage hard conversations with my mom and dad. To their credit, they listened well, receiving these exchanges as opportunities to mature.

It's not wrong or disrespectful to ask hard questions of your life, or even of your parents. In Scripture, King Hezekiah had to ponder the abuses of his father in a massive reckoning that shook the very foundations of that society (2 Kings 18). My children—now grown and married—have called me out on my own contradictions, quite courageously given that I teach these things for a living.

Perhaps we honor our parents and the generations before us best when we become truth tellers, and in so doing, pave the path to becoming ourselves. One way to begin that process is to consider the consequences when our core needs for attachment and authenticity go unmet. There are different pathways this can take: disowned authenticity, performative authenticity, or chaotic authenticity.

Disowned Authenticity

A first pathway is the cultivation of attachment without authenticity. This often results in enmeshed children. Unwittingly tethered to their parents' needs and expectations, they are unfamiliar with their own inner terrain and unique inscape. Their identity forms around the fragile ecosystem of external approval, resulting in perpetual insecurity and anxiety—adults chasing a sense of self but never feeling like themselves.

Years ago I counseled Angela, a woman who was trained by her mother in a particular vision of womanhood. Her mother told her that she'd eventually be old enough to get married and have babies, thus fulfilling her purpose in life. The rooting she'd need, she was told, was in a Christian man.

When it came time for college, Angela was sent off to a Christian university to find a husband and fulfill her destiny as wife, mother, and homemaker. A small and relentless voice within her wanted something different, but she learned to suppress it. At one point, she dared to declare that she'd like to be an art major, but she was told in no uncertain terms that she'd need to choose a major with classes filled with eligible Christian bachelors, apparently not the kinds of boys you'd find in art classes.

"What you want doesn't matter," her mother said. "God's will is what matters." Angela's mom was unattuned to God's unique design within her daughter, his creative longing for her life.

Angela quietly nurtured her love for art, drawing late at night. Eventually, she did meet a man, get married, and fulfill the expectations of her parents. But in her midthirties she grew depressed, which her physician treated as a serotonin issue until a wise friend said, "Angela, this isn't about a broken brain. This is grief."[4]

"It cost me so much to live someone else's image of who I should be," she told me. "I was clamoring for my mother's approval. I was living her ideal of a life. But I wasn't living mine."

This is the first pathway that diverts so many people from living out their true inscape. Like many people, Angela grew up with a sense of attachment, but not authenticity. She was so tied to her parents' hopes and dreams that she had no connection to her own inner self, ignoring her deepest desires to meet her family's expectations. Everything about her identity formed around the fragile ecosystem of external approval, resulting in perpetual insecurity and anxiety. She had spent her life chasing a sense of self but never feeling quite like she'd ever been herself.

Performative Authenticity

A second pathway is the cultivation of authenticity without attachment. This often results in isolation and autonomy—but a tenuous autonomy. People may pride themselves on self-sufficiency but carry an underground ache of disconnection. They may project a sense of confidence or externally parade their authenticity, but feel unmoored within—adults who struggle to trust, connect, and rest in the presence of another. This leads to performative authenticity.

Jordan, the social media influencer you met at the start of the chapter, was killing time in an airport, scrolling absentmindedly, when one of his own videos appeared in his feed—an older clip he'd forgotten about. He watched it the way one watches a stranger. The pauses were calibrated. The vulnerability timed. Even the sigh before he spoke felt rehearsed.

Halfway through, Jordan felt a tightening in his chest.

Who is this? he thought. It was the first time he recognized his own forced authenticity.

Shame washed over him—a shame that motivated him to reach out. Our work together honored the genuine shift he was trying to make from his father's polished certainty toward something more honest, raw, and messy. Slowly, Jordan named the deeper ache beneath the performance: that he'd rarely been seen, that he was searching for a mirror that could reflect his worth without requiring him to perform for it.

Learning to receive that kind of reflection without an audience became the quiet work of his healing.

Chaotic Authenticity

A third pathway is the absence of both attachment and authenticity. Here, a child internalizes a sense of profound abandonment—both from others and from self. Because they feel neither seen nor cherished by their parents or caregivers, they may experience pervasive shame, a fragmented identity, emotional dysregulation, and internalized self-rejection. Their inner narrative often sounds like, *I am alone. I am wrong. I am nothing.* In adulthood, this can manifest as relational dysfunction (clinging, avoiding, grasping, attention seeking) or chronically self-destructive patterns (addiction, dissociation, self-harm). This leads to the push-pull of both disowned and performative authenticity, resulting in a kind of chaotic authenticity.

Megan often felt like she was either too much or not enough, sometimes within the same hour. She'd reach for connection impulsively, then recoil in shame, unsure what she'd done wrong. This is what she'd done since her earliest days—hoping her busy single mom might eventually notice her but often experiencing a beating when she sought her attention.

The story Megan carried was simple and merciless: *I am not loved, and I have nothing to offer.* What emerged in adulthood was fragmentation—raw self-exposure followed by collapse, grasping followed by withdrawal. It looked chaotic on the outside, but it was the logic of survival in a life formed without love or affirmation.

THREE FACES OF FRAGMENTED AUTHENTICITY

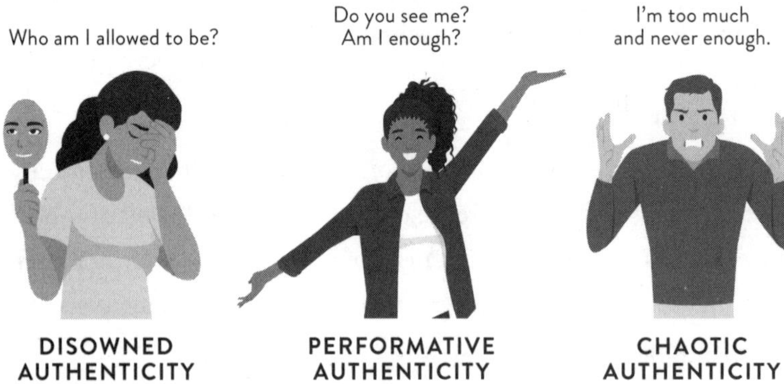
Who am I allowed to be?
Do you see me?
Am I enough?
I'm too much
and never enough.
DISOWNED
AUTHENTICITY
PERFORMATIVE
AUTHENTICITY
CHAOTIC
AUTHENTICITY

All three forms of fragmented authenticity are recipes for character shaped not merely in dysregulation but also in rootlessness—leading to inner division, insecurity, and inauthenticity. I'm somewhere in that mix, and I suspect some of you reading right now might be too.

Some of us live with a buzzing envy within, quietly coveting a friend's job, a colleague's success, an influencer's shining personality. Some of us have climbed the ladder to perceived success, only to find we still feel empty. Some of us are resigned to a sense of shame and despair. But I sense a deep longing for more in so many people

I talk to—a desire for rootedness in a stable and secure self, despite the pull of the digital egosphere to perform authenticity.

Thomas Merton sensed this decades ago:

> There is in us an instinct for newness, for renewal, for a liberation of creative power. We seek to awaken in ourselves a force which really changes our lives from within. And yet the same instinct tells us that this change is a recovery of that which is deepest, most original, most personal in ourselves. To be born again is not to become somebody else, *but to become ourselves.*[5]

There isn't an exact equation to become ourselves, though I wish there were. What I do know is that this process must begin with honesty.

Awakening to Our Inscape

Rooted Repentance

The apostle Paul prayed that the church in Ephesus would be "rooted and grounded in love" (Ephesians 3:17, ESV), and it's this secure foundation that allows us to be our true selves in a world of anxiety, envy, greed, jealousy, and acquisitiveness. This is the kind of rooted authenticity that makes for strong friendships, connected marriages, healthy systems, grounded leaders, and creative work. This is the kind of rooted authenticity that grows character.

But this can take time, particularly when we've disowned or chased after authenticity. Too often, I've seen fauxnerability used as an attempted shortcut—a kind of rootless repentance that performs apologies and postures with apparently sincere words, all the while sidestepping real confession. I'm old enough to remember televangelist Jimmy Swaggart's tearful sermon in 1988 amidst a sex scandal. "I have sinned," he said, tears flowing and voice quivering. Three months later, however, he was back in the pulpit with more tears, proclaiming, "Guilt is not of God. . . . I will never again look back."[6] He later launched a Christian television network.

"You mean, I have to step away from doing what God has called me to do?" said one pastor, after I told him he'd need to leave the platform to find himself. He did step down, but not three months into our counseling work, he'd already started a podcast. "I'm just itchy if I don't have an outlet for my teachings," he said.

I told him he'd have to live with the itch a whole lot longer.

The instinct makes sense: When your authentic voice has been squelched, you have little access to a core capacity for true confession. Before a person can offer a genuine confession or apology, they need time to dismantle the old disowned or performative self, and to find their own voice (Ephesians 4:22-24). Anything less makes for a cheap confession. Fast fixes, accelerated apologies, and quick comebacks aren't helpful; if you've been harmed, you ought to expect nothing less than a sincere confession. But you might have to wait a long, long time for it.

As I've worked in spaces of narcissism and abuse for nearly three decades, I've noticed that apologies deepen when people do the inner work of dismantling old character architecture. But we can't rush this process. We can't perform our way back to health or wholeness, and we certainly can't fake deep character change.

Faithful Formation

Years ago when I was dismantling old, weary parts of me that attempted to perform my way to academic success and spiritual leadership, I heard something that stuck with me. Someone described the fruit of the spirit of "faithfulness" in a new way—as a *fidelity*, not to the many oughts and shoulds around me but to God's unique image and workmanship within me. In her poem "The Journey," Mary Oliver speaks to the clamoring voices around you that demand things—the voices that beckon you to perform, to conform, to rescue, to succeed, to master, to perfect. But the hope is that as you leave these anxious voices behind, you'll discover,

> *there was a new voice*
> *which you slowly*
> *recognized as your own.*[7]

And so I learned to listen within, more carefully and with more kindness. At first, my mentor Gary sat with me as I learned to listen. And then Roger. And then Gordon, And then Jay. Each played a vital role in mentoring me into my depths. With growing fidelity to that new and true voice, something began to shift inside me. I first learned to listen to, then to love, this new, emerging voice. With growing inner attention, my habits began to shift from fauxnerability to fidelity. Slowly, they became automaticities—second nature—new habits of a maturing heart.

As St. Augustine (354–430) said long ago, "Gather yourself together into your real self."[8]

The process hasn't come without setbacks—it's tough to leave the old voices behind. At times, it feels like it's taking too long. At other times still, I wonder if I have anything meaningful to offer.

Shifting the architecture of our character is a lifelong endeavor.

But it's worth it.

In a world of performative authenticity and fauxnerability, we'll need to slow down and sort through words offered amidst haste, hustle, and hubris. We'll have to sift through faux apologies, perhaps even AI-generated confessions today.

But beneath it all—if we're willing to see—is the *poiēma*, the exquisitely imaged, divinely designed you. And me. The Christian inscape tradition suggests that real character formation is not about chasing after an abstract conception outside yourself, but about reclaiming a God-implanted design for goodness, beauty, and truth within. This formation process is not a performance but an unfolding, an uncovering of the deepest truth about who we are—living icons of God's image, God's poetic workmanship (Ephesians 2:10; Colossians 3:9-10).

We're not just trusting ourselves or some vague gut intuition; we're trusting that we're designed for worth, for belonging, and for purpose—three core aspects of God's image in us. And we're trusting that we serve the world best not when we disown our authenticity or perform it, but when we're deeply connected to ourselves and thus connected to a larger story God is writing through us.

We'll have to work for it and wait for it.

We'll have to sift through all the counterfeit voices within and without that might seek to unroot our authentic selves, just as the serpent did in Genesis 3.

Yet in time, the "rooted and grounded" you and I will emerge, charting a new course, transforming the very architecture of our character, cultivating a true authenticity.

So, dear friends,

May you have the courage to grow downward,
to root yourself not in performance or applause,

but in the sacred soil of your true self—
the image of God uniquely woven into you.

May the old voices lose their grip,
and may the voice that is yours alone rise with quiet confidence.
Not curated. Not performed. But true.

And when the world tempts you to perform what should be lived,
may you choose fidelity over fauxnerability,
depth over display,
integrity over imitation.

May you become who you are—
not in haste, but in holy patience—
as the poiēma *of God emerges in you, word by living word.*

RESOURCES

- Gabor Maté, *The Myth of Normal: Trauma, Illness, and Healing in a Toxic Culture*
- Thomas Merton, *New Seeds of Contemplation*
- Mary Oliver, *New and Selected Poems, Volume One*
- David Whyte, *The Poetry of Self-Compassion* (audio)

REFLECTION

1. As you consider your own story, can you name someone in your life who helped you discover the authentic you? Did someone who loved you help you listen to the inner melody line that is uniquely yours—and live it out—with confidence? If so, explain.

2. If your parent or caregiver did not help you live into your authentic self, can you sense the loss that comes from being disconnected from this deeper you? In what ways has this led you to feel as if you have to perform, wear a mask, or become what others need you to become?
3. How have you seen fauxnerability play out in your life? In the life of others?
4. Which factors at play in a life where you're cut off from your innate authenticity can you relate to? How did they impact you in the long run, personally and relationally?
5. How does recognizing that you are God's image bearer with a unique inscape, created to be a particular kind of presence in the world, affect you? What might change if you were seen for who you really are?
6. As you ponder disowned, performative, and chaotic authenticity (see pages 59–62), which one do you relate to the most? How has it played out personally and relationally?
7. Repentance and change come at a cost. They are slow. They are hard. But they return you to a rootedness you were designed and created for by a God who sees you at the core and who loves what he sees. Imagine you could live from here on being seen and known, in a way that requires less struggle and more freedom. How might your life be different if you lived like this?

PRACTICE

Cultivating Feeling Seen for the Sake of Character Change

Curt Thompson writes, "We all are born into the world looking for someone looking for us, and that we remain in this mode of searching for the rest of our lives."[9] Feeling seen provides the deep recognition our nervous systems and souls need in order to let down our guard. When someone reflects back our worth, our uniqueness, and even our wounds with compassion rather than judgment, our defenses relax, and the internal exile of the hidden parts of ourselves begins to end. In that relational light, we can finally stop performing, tell the truth about ourselves, and enter the vulnerable spaces where character formation is enabled.

STEP 1: SEEK TO BE SEEN

We all desperately long to be seen. The question is: Who really sees you? It's crucial that you find people in your life who can (a) bear witness to who you are at your created core and (b) bear witness to you amidst the wounds you've inflicted and/or received. Consider your story. Was there a parent, grandparent, caregiver, coach, teacher, mentor, babysitter, or pastor who really saw you? What did it feel like? Simply dwell for a few minutes in the feeling of being seen.

Now consider your present-day experience. Is there someone who really sees you? Is there someone who can both bear witness to your beauty and worth, and even to the way you've sinned against others or been sinned against? Is there someone who sees you with your wounds and doesn't look away? If not, might there be someone you can ask to enter into this sacred space with you—a therapist, mentor, pastor, or spiritual director?

STEP 2: RELAX IN THE PRESENCE OF GOD

We can also engage embodied practices of feeling seen, even by God. It's important to find a quiet, unhurried space where you can simply relax into your own presence, reconnecting with yourself in body and soul, and rest in the presence of the divine.

- Relax and breathe gently, placing your hands on your cheeks.
- If it seems right to you, hear God whispering, "I long to make my face shine upon you and be gracious to you" (see Numbers 6:24-26).

- Turn this ancient blessing into a breath prayer if it helps:

  (Inhale) God, you long to bless me and keep me,

  (Exhale) To shine your face upon me and be gracious to me,

  (Inhale) To show me your favor

  (Exhale) And give me your peace.

- Close your eyes and imagine a smile of delight from Jesus, or if you'd prefer, the smile of a friend or mentor, a spouse or partner.
- As you sense your body relaxing, you might whisper to yourself, "I am seen. I am delighted in. I can relax and reconnect."

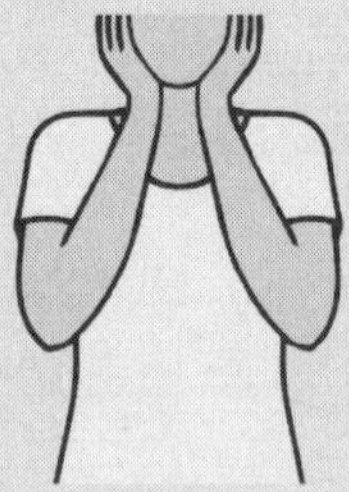

SEEN

Feeling seen is an antidote to a primal shame that might have been mapped in your earliest years—a shame that orients your character toward self-protection or prompts you to chase influence, platform, power, or attention.

To be seen is to be mirrored by another with compassion and kindness, opening yourself to be known at the deepest level and freeing you from the exhausting chase for acceptance. Your character is best shaped to produce the fruit of love, joy, peace, patience, kindness, goodness, faithfulness, gentleness, and self-control when your defenses relax, your heart opens, and you experience feeling both safe and seen.

CHAPTER 3

reflective

Seeking the Right Kind of Attention

Attention is the beginning of devotion.
MARY OLIVER

We all, who with unveiled faces contemplate the Lord's glory, are being transformed into his image with ever-increasing glory, which comes from the Lord, who is the Spirit.
2 CORINTHIANS 3:18

Jamie was born in 1999 and raised online. By middle school, his worldview was already being shaped not by mentors or embodied community but by algorithmic currents—feeds filled with hot takes and truth bombs. He was discipled in a digital catechesis that rewarded reactivity over reflection, certainty over curiosity, and ideation over integrity.

By the time he entered a midwestern Christian college, Jamie had a growing platform as a Christian cultural commentator. His gift was clarity, or at least the appearance of it. He could articulate the "biblical view" on anything from sexuality to economics in five hundred characters or less on X and Truth Social. He prided himself on being bold and unafraid to "stand for truth in a compromising age."

His phone rarely left his hand. He lived in the dopamine feedback loop of outrage and affirmation, endlessly reacting to the next story, calling out the next heresy, seizing the next moment for likes. He was always on—his attention fractured, his soul restless.

What he couldn't yet name was that the world that taught him to be *right* had never taught him to be *present*.

Jamie had been formed—spiritually, neurologically, culturally—by a world that confused attention with affection and reactivity with righteousness. His character, though seemingly sharp on the surface, was thin and brittle beneath. What he didn't admit online was that he rarely slept well. That he lived with a low-grade anxiety that never quite left his chest. That his relationships were mostly transactional. That he felt disconnected from his own body, not to mention from God. And though he still posted daily and debated endlessly, a quiet ache had begun to form within him, like questions with no audience:

Who am I without the likes?
What remains when the scrolling stops?

Dopamine Seeking

Jamie's story reflects life in an addictive digital economy, one predicated on capturing and keeping attention. Attention isn't just scattered—it's *commodified.*

What's the result?

This creates, not just distraction, but spiritual fragmentation—a slow erosion of our integrity and our capacity for connection, rootedness, and sustained attention. As my friend and global ecumenical leader Wes Granberg-Michaelson points out, this attention economy doesn't just distract us—it forms us.[1] He notes that this is precisely what C. S. Lewis foresaw in *The Screwtape Letters*: the demonic strategy of keeping souls disengaged, preoccupied, and numb.[2]

We work to excess. We lose ourselves in mindless entertainment. We click from headline to headline. We eat away our emptiness. We scroll our way into promises of better bodies and less stress. We whisper about the latest friend drama. We caffeinate our mornings and medicate away the churning anxiety at night with a few too many drinks.

When we're always chasing the next dopamine surge of (temporary) glory, life becomes a mindless and exhausting hunt after our next fix, quite literally. What we're actually seeking is neurochemical—a dopamine high, which fills us with nearly instantaneous but fleeting feelings of pleasure. In the end, our nervous systems are shaped toward reactivity, primed for digital warfare, and rendered incapable of sustained presence. All of this shapes our character.

In her bestselling book *Dopamine Nation*, Anna Lembke explains that constantly chasing the next dopamine hit actually undermines our capacity for joy and satisfaction in life.[3] When we overindulge in pleasurable activities—whether it's social media, sugar, sex, or shopping—we tip the brain's delicate balance of pleasure and pain toward a chronic state of dissatisfaction. This triggers the brain's homeostatic response, lowering our baseline dopamine levels and making ordinary life feel dull, even heightening our anxiety in the long run.

The more we pursue instant gratification, she says, the more we desensitize ourselves to it—requiring even more stimulation just to feel "normal." Eventually, our habitual patterns erode our sense of self-control, ultimately making us feel less resilient, less present, and less able to enjoy life. And this isn't just the plight of the so-called addict who can't shake alcohol or gambling—this is each of us embedded within this attention economy.

Of course, for most of us, we didn't wake up one day and choose this. A thousand little mindless choices formed us in a particular way, shaping our character.

"The first mistake is never the one that ruins you," writes James Clear in his bestselling book *Atomic Habits*. "It is the spiral of repeated mistakes that follows. Missing once is an accident. Missing twice is the start of a new habit."[4]

And, as we know, our habits tell the story of who we are and what we love.

Habits of Disconnection

"I woke up one day and realized I wasn't alive," Cheryl said, holding back sobs. "I looked back ten, even twenty years, and saw a blur. I wasn't living."

"I wondered why I was so depressed even though I had the life, the job, and the family I'd wanted," Harry said. "And then I realized it wasn't my life I was living."

When we're dysregulated within and out of touch with our unique inscape, we become unmoored, untethered, adrift at sea. I've worked with people earning six- and seven-figure incomes whose lives looked like success stories but who felt utterly lost, disconnected within, creatures of heart-habits that had become their unfortunate norm.

When we finally do awaken from our stupor, whether through a dramatic event like a public failure or just a gnawing and growing sense that something isn't right, we may be stunned as we reflect on our habits and realize how entrenched they have become.

Brain researcher and best-selling author Joe Dispenza writes

> We are creatures of habit. We think somewhere between 60,000 to 70,000 thoughts in one day, and 90 percent of those thoughts are exactly the same ones we had the day before. We get up on the same side of the bed, go through the same routine in the bathroom, comb our hair in the same way, sit in the same chair as we eat the same breakfast and hold our mug in the same hand, drive the same route to the same job, and do the same things we know how to do so well with the same people (who push the same emotional buttons) every day. And then we hurry up and go home so that we can hurry up and check our e-mail so that we can hurry up and eat dinner so that we can hurry up and watch our favorite TV shows so that we can hurry up and brush our teeth in the same bedtime routine so that we can hurry up and go to bed at the same time so that we can hurry up and do it all over again the next day. If it sounds as though I'm saying that we live a huge part of our lives on autopilot, that's exactly right.[5]

And when we become creatures of unreflective habits, these patterns may come to define our most important relationships and activities. Life on autopilot begins to be characterized by certain symptoms:

- *Emotional numbness:* By not paying attention to your inner world, you lose any meaningful contact to your longings, your grief, your hope, your joy.
- *Performative spirituality:* You attend church, read Scripture, or perhaps even pray—but without interior engagement.

Eventually, your spiritual life feels empty and stagnant, marked more by conformity than by communion.

- *Marital stagnation:* You move through life side by side but no longer face-to-face. Routines replace intimacy, conversations become transactional, and tenderness gives way to efficiency. The relationship may look fine on the surface, but beneath it lies a quiet ache: a loss of curiosity, play, and deep knowing.
- *Unattuned parenting:* You might respond to your child's emotions with clichés ("You're fine," "Get over it") rather than curiosity. Over time, this can teach children to hide their feelings, and it can shape you into a disconnected, dismissive parent rather than an attuned one.
- *Numbing routines of consumption:* You open your phone, the fridge, or a streaming service whenever discomfort arises. These habits become a familiar escape route. This trains your brain to reach for a dopamine hit, avoiding the very growth discomfort offers.
- *Conflict avoidance in close relationships:* When you repeatedly choose silence over hard conversations, you may preserve surface peace but forfeit the deeper trust that only honesty builds. Over time, you are shaped into a peacekeeper rather than a peacemaker.

Yes, you are a creature of habit. And so am I. Habits are, in fact, inviolably human. You can't avoid habits. But you can begin to reflect on them and, in so doing, reshape your character.

Reflection Reshapes Us

This call to (self) reflection is another ancient gift of the Christian tradition. In his *Confessions*, St. Augustine spends nine chapters reflecting on his life, confessing his divided attention and returning to the one who'd been pursuing him all the while. It was Augustine who gave me—a biblical studies guy skeptical of the therapeutic—the courage to begin looking at my own life.

Reflection invites us to ask ourselves, *What do I give my attention to?*

If we're honest, we're a lot like Augustine—our loves divided, our lives inattentive. We awaken to our lives, as the poet Mary Oliver notes in her lovely book *Upstream*, sensing that we've been lost in a sea of distraction and that we're being called to renewed attunement and attention:

> With growth into adulthood, responsibilities claimed me, so many heavy coats. I didn't choose them, I don't fault them, but it took time to reject them. Now in the spring I kneel, I put my face into the packets of violets, the dampness, the freshness, the sense of ever-ness. Something is wrong, I know it, if I don't keep my attention on eternity.

She sums up this shift beautifully, writing, "Attention is the beginning of devotion."[6]

Oliver awakened in adulthood to the reality that she'd lost touch with her soul, with the earth, even with a sense of eternity. She was asking questions each of us might ask: *What do I love? What do I give my heart to? Where do I place my attention, and thus my devotion?*

How might you answer those questions?

At a retreat not long ago, I asked the participants to reflect on their heart-habits. Then I posed the question: What do these habits reveal about what you love?

If you would have asked them beforehand, they might have said,

"I love God. I cherish my closest relationships. I long to contribute to the world meaningfully and generously." But after this exercise, they were astounded by their divided loves, by their inner contradictions.

A retreat participant named Eileen was honest in her self-assessment: "My habits reveal something quite different than the idealized version of myself I came in with. The themes I discovered are embarrassing to admit, but that's the only way forward. So here's my honest answer—my habits reveal that I love convenience, comfort, consumption, control, and covetousness. I've devoted my heart, even my attention, to chasing these things."

Mind you, Eileen was a church elder and someone thought to be wise, disciplined, and consistent. And yet like so many of us, her hidden contradictions were a surprise to her.

Honest self-reflection awakens your powers of attention, activating your DLPFC, or dorsolateral prefrontal cortex, the region in the brain primarily involved in executive functions and cognitive control. Psychiatrist Curt Thompson names it the brain's spotlight, inviting you and me to pay attention to what we're paying attention to.[7] For Eileen and others, this shift from assumption to attention is a crucial one, awakening us to the neurobiological possibility of deep change.

The Power of Imagination

What we behold, we become.[8]

When our attention is shaped by a need for others to see us—even through our performative spirituality—our character conforms. And there is no character change without a significant shift in attention.

Steven Garber, author and founder of the Washington Institute for Faith, Vocation and Culture, names this dynamic: "Day by day we are forming characters and forming cultures in the way we respond to the world. If we are to avoid the paralysis of destructive cynicism and debilitating sorrow, somehow, somewhere, we have to make sense of the world—not only of our own lives, but of life."[9]

We now know that this "making sense of life" begins with attention. You see, what we give our attention to quite literally *shapes the architecture of our brains*—and over time, our character. And imagination is the key to focusing our attention.

For so many of us, our imaginations have been hijacked. We wake up in midlife, like Mary Oliver did, wondering who we are and what has become of our lives. It takes attuned self-reflection coupled with a renewed imagination to begin shaping the kind of life we long for.

The now well-known neuroscientific insight that "neurons that fire together, wire together" applies: Repeated focus on certain thoughts, emotions, or behaviors strengthens the neural pathways that support them. (We'll practice this in chapter 8.) When our attention is directed toward self-protection or performance, power or persona, it reinforces patterns of anxiety and disconnection. That leads us to perpetual Storm or Fog. But when we cultivate our attention with curiosity and openness, longing and hope, it creates space for transformation, allowing us to be reshaped by love, connection, coherence, and presence.

I think of a friend of mine who had gotten into the habit of picking up her phone as soon as she woke up each morning. She recognized that she'd long been habituated to anxious coping and that this act reinforced that. As she began to cultivate safety within, her heart softened, and she noticed a desire to start her mornings in quiet meditation. She didn't force a new habit—rather, an emerging sense of safety and feeling seen by God shifted something within. Her developing imagination and longing for gentle mornings rather than anxious ones grew. Sometimes she practiced a body scan, attuning to her embodied senses to notice the world around her. At other times, she imagined herself peacefully sitting on her favorite beach, Jesus by her side. Later she noted how much more grounded she felt throughout the day because of this fundamental shift.

True character formation requires intentional attention—deciding to use practices that retune our thoughts, regulate our nervous systems, and restore healthy relationships.

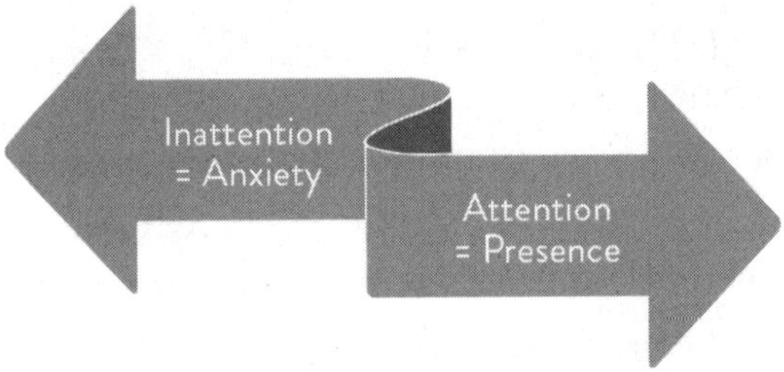

There is no real character change absent a deepening of your attention.

I've seen a simple shift in myself over the last few years, largely due to my wife's prompting. Sara sees beauty in ways I don't, and she sees it specifically—in the kinds of trees that stretch their arms in praise in our backyard; or in the goldfinch, with its bright yellow plumage, singing sweetly even as it bounces through the air.

I sat in our yard one afternoon a few years back, my phone tucked away, and simply gazed for a while, allowing my senses to be retuned.

And I began to see.

With my imagination expanding, I began to deliberately pay attention to our winged visitors in the days after, how the white-breasted nuthatch forages headfirst down tree trunks, defying gravity with ease. How the red-headed woodpecker hammers bark in search of insects.

Strangely, now I see.

And what's more, my brain has been reshaped to spot a particular kind of beauty—in birds—something I couldn't have said a few years back. I can honestly say that my loves have shifted—that I *love* birdwatching. Moreover, I now see beauty in a way I wasn't able to before, given my inattention. It's a simple example, and yet a powerful story of how we can change not only our minds but our loves as well.

What might you learn by paying attention to what you're paying attention to? How might this reveal what your heart loves, what it's devoted to? And how might this practice begin to reshape not just your brain, but your character?

N. T. Wright, who offers a theological take on this neurobiological phenomenon, notes how character is shaped amidst our choices:

> Virtue . . . is what happens when someone has made a thousand small choices, requiring effort and concentration, to do something which is good and right but which doesn't "come naturally"—and then, on the thousand and first time, when it really matters, they find that they do what's required "automatically." . . . *Virtue* is what happens when wise and courageous choices have become "second nature."[10]

I agree, but with a caveat.

While it's true that character is shaped through small, repeated decisions, we too often overlook the soil in which those choices are planted. Real, lasting change—as we've seen—rarely takes root in a nervous system locked in survival mode.

The Virtues of Attention-Seeking

Even with good practices and worthy intentions, someone trapped in a self-protective survival state will remain stuck. I've seen it time and again. But I've also witnessed the dynamics of deep change.

As I was preparing for an extended counseling intensive with a pastor accused of grandiosity, entitlement, and attention-seeking, I interviewed several of his staff members, asking them to provide personal narratives of their experiences. The pastor came in resistant, in survival mode, hopeful for a quick comeback story and my seal of approval. Instead, our work together was marked by a close reading of the narratives I'd collected, a process that seemed quite painful to my client.

And yet our days together softened him. He began to feel safe with me, his countenance relaxing, his eyes becoming gentle, his words growing more aligned, more honest. Here, out of the spotlight, he was beginning to feel known. He started to lay down his defenses and accept the harm he'd done.

After a lengthy session with me, he spent the evening reflecting on his heart's habits, the orientation and direction of his loves. When he returned the next morning, I noticed his eyes, puffed and pink at the edges, bearing the weight of a night's worth of weeping. He sat down and showed me a letter of resignation he'd written to his church, with the beginnings of an apology and a promise to do whatever work he needed to do to understand his impact.

And then he asked if he could read me a passage that he'd read the night before, lines from Fyodor Dostoevsky's *The Brothers Karamazov*:

> Above all, avoid falsehood, every kind of falsehood, especially falseness to yourself. Watch over your own deceitfulness and look into it every hour, every minute. Avoid being scornful, both to others and to yourself. What seems to you bad within you will grow purer from the very fact of your observing it in yourself. Avoid fear, too, though fear is only the consequence of every sort of falsehood. Never be frightened at your own faint-heartedness in attaining love. Don't be frightened overmuch even at your evil actions. . . . I predict that just when you see with horror that in spite of all your efforts you are getting farther from your goal instead of nearer to it—at that very moment I predict that you will reach it and behold clearly the miraculous power of the Lord who has been all the time loving and mysteriously guiding you.[11]

The last line evoked more tears, his heart's deepest longing for love revealed.

His story was like so many I hear.

His mother praised tidiness but offered no touch; his father demanded excellence but withheld warmth. So he learned to earn affection by becoming exceptional, curating a persona that masked his hunger for real connection. By middle school, he had mastered the art of performance—winning awards, commanding attention, charming adults, all the while stuck in survival mode.

But beneath the polish lived a quiet ache, a terror of being unseen. He buried that fear under layers of charisma, wit, and control.

Over time, he came to believe that if he stopped shining, he might disappear altogether.

His narcissism wasn't born from vanity—it was born from absence. From a heart that repeatedly reached out and was not met, from eyes that gazed with longing, only to find that no one was looking back.

What this pastor longed for—and what each of us needs—is safety, connection, a loving gaze. Until a person feels safe, physiologically and relationally, new habits can't flourish. It is within the safety of secure connection, where we are seen, soothed, and supported, that the brain and nervous system begin to quiet their defenses and the soul dares to choose differently.

The morning that pastor read the Dostoevsky passage to me is one I won't soon forget. He felt safe enough to be held in his tears, something he'd not experienced before. It would take years for his attachments to become secure and for his character to be reshaped. But it would come through the safety of relationship—with me, but also with God, who as Dostoevsky says, "has been all the time loving and mysteriously guiding you."

C. S. Lewis also understood this, writing that God "has infinite attention to spare for each one of us. . . . You are as much alone with Him as if you were the only being He had ever created."[12]

Attachment is not a footnote to transformation—it is its foundation.

Seen and Soothed

This is the ironic intent of attention-seeking—the longing to be seen and known.

"I've been preaching about God's love for years, but I've never felt it," pastors tell me, over and over again. Most of them also confess that they were never apprenticed in contemplative prayer practices and rarely stop long enough for an encounter with God.

Remember Jamie, whose identity was formed through digital discipleship? Tech addiction is an obvious problem for many people today, but C. S. Lewis reminds us that distraction can come in many forms and in any era. As Screwtape observes, habits eventually make what once offered pleasure less effective yet harder to give up:

> You no longer need a good book, which he really likes, to keep him from his prayers or his work or his sleep; a column of advertisements in yesterday's paper will do. You can make him waste his time not only in conversation he enjoys with people whom he likes, but in conversations with those he cares nothing about on subjects that bore him. . . . You will say that these are very small sins; and doubtless, like all young tempters, you are anxious to be able to report spectacular wickedness. But do remember, the only thing that matters is the extent to which you separate the man from the Enemy [God].[13]

In his *Confessions*, Augustine spends nine chapters reflecting on his own distraction and division. He then offers one of the most beautiful expositions of a scattered heart finding its true security once again:

> Late have I loved you, beauty so old and so new: late have I loved you. And see, you were within and I was in the external world and sought you there, and in my unlovely state I plunged into those lovely created things which you made. You were with me, and I was not with you. The lovely things kept

> me far from you, though if they did not have their existence in you, they had no existence at all. You called and cried out loud and shattered my deafness. You were radiant and resplendent, you put to flight my blindness. You were fragrant, and I drew in my breath and now pant after you. I tasted you, and I feel but hunger and thirst for you. You touched me, and I am set on fire to attain the peace which is yours.[14]

Augustine chased that feeling of being seen by others and soothed in his addictions for years. Yet, amidst his inattention and restlessness, secure love created the heart conditions for substantial change. Secure love awakened new hungers that led to new habits that, in the end, soothed his dysregulated soul and shifted his character. The prodigal of passion became a pilgrim of presence.

When we lift our eyes to behold the face of Christ, something deep within us begins to change—not through striving, but through sustained attention to the one who sees us fully and loves us still. It is in the act of contemplation, of turning toward God's radiant presence with unveiled faces, as 2 Corinthians 3:16 reminds us, that we are gradually transformed. When we're seen in this way, something relaxes within—we're soothed at the deepest level. Here, the anxious chase can end and true security can grow.

This is the birthplace of character change.

"Can people really change?" I'm often asked. As we're seeing, there is no easy path. Sadly, the transformative path we're offered is often yet another series of things to do, ways to keep busy, or things to fill our minds with. Rarely are we offered the slow path, the one where we still ourselves long enough to be seen and soothed, satiating the deep hunger within.

This transformation is not self-manufactured but Spirit-wrought, a reshaping of our character from the inside out. In the gaze of God, we come home to ourselves—more whole, more free, more Christlike.

To live under that gaze is to become, in time, what we were always meant to be. To become ourselves.

And so, dear friends,

May you grow weary of the chase,
the endless striving to be noticed,
the restless reaching for the next fix of fleeting glory.

May you see what it's cost you:
your presence, your peace, your truest self.

And may something deeper awaken in you—
a holy ache,
a longing not to be impressive,
but to be seen . . . and still loved.

May you come to trust the gaze of the one
who has always been looking your way—
not to critique, but to cherish,
not to measure, but to mend.

May this love quiet the noise.
May it soothe your soul.
May it reshape your habits.
And may it root you,
again and again,
in the grace that never looks away.

RESOURCES

- Augustine, *Confessions*
- Anna Lembke, *Dopamine Nation: Finding Balance in the Age of Indulgence*
- Curt Thompson, *Anatomy of the Soul: Surprising Connections Between Neuroscience and Spiritual Practices That Can Transform Your Life and Relationships*
- N. T. Wright, *After You Believe: Why Christian Character Matters*

REFLECTION

1. Your heart and habits have been shaped in a particular way over time. What is the story of how your heart and habits were formed?
2. Reflect on where your attention goes when you're living on autopilot. Each of us seeks a kind of soothing, even if we're unaware of it. If we are honest about our hearts and habits, we can admit that we may seek soothing in various ways: in inordinate attention or affection from others, in substances, in scrolling social media or binge-watching television, perhaps even in things that look religious or righteous. What do your habits reveal about where your attention goes and how you self-soothe?
3. As you reflect on your story and your current habits, can you name the roots of your inattention and self-soothing? When you were growing up, what was missing? How did you learn to calm yourself even at an early age? What was modeled for you?
4. What longings grow in you as you consider the kind of person you want to be? How would your habits and heart be different if you lived the kind of life you were made for?
5. How do you experience the presence of God? Do you feel safe, seen, and soothed in his presence? Can you rest there? It's okay

if your story is one in which God didn't feel safe or caring—that's a common experience. If that's how you felt, do you long for something different? How would you articulate your heart's longing in words, perhaps even in a prayer?

PRACTICE

Examining Your Habits and Longings for the Sake of Character Change

Most of us live unaware of our inner dysregulation, but we frequently act on it—our bodies chasing dopamine hits to provide some hint of self-soothing. These habits shape our character. We look for a bit of neurochemical comfort in too much food or alcohol, in pornography or compulsive sex, in chronic overwork, in endless scrolling, in impulse shopping, spending, and gambling, even in humor or sarcasm. These, in time, become habits of the heart.

But a deeper peace is available. And as you experience feeling safe, seen, and soothed, your defenses relax, your longings awaken, and you discover a connection to what is deepest and truest within. You awaken to the created goodness of your image-bearing self, even the sacred desires of your Spirit-led self.

If "attention is the beginning of devotion," as Mary Oliver says, consider what your everyday practices reveal about where you seek comfort.

1. Reflect on your habits. What do they reveal about what you give your attention to and how you practice self-soothing?
2. What do these habits reveal about what you love?
3. Next shift your attention to your longings, completing this sentence:

   My deepest desire is to become a person who . . .

   ____

   ____

As you begin to ponder this final part of the exercise, consider the following biblical texts, which invite this new form of attention:

> The human spirit is the lamp of the LORD
>   that sheds light on one's inmost being.
>
> PROVERBS 20:27

> We all, who with unveiled faces contemplate the Lord's glory, are being transformed into his image with ever-increasing glory, which comes from the Lord, who is the Spirit.
>
> 2 CORINTHIANS 3:18

PRACTICE

Cultivating Feeling Soothed for the Sake of Character Change

Now awaken to a deeper soothing that is available if you're willing to shift your attention and relax your defenses. You can experience feeling safe and seen by those who love you, by God, and even within yourself. Let's practice this as you offer an inner attentiveness from your core, true self to the parts of you that feel anxious, chaotic, and even unseen.

STEP 1: SELF-SOOTHE THROUGH BREATHWORK

Gently breathe, placing your nondominant hand on your chest, moving it slowly and tenderly in a circular motion. Whisper within to every wounded and weary part of yourself, "Ssshhh."

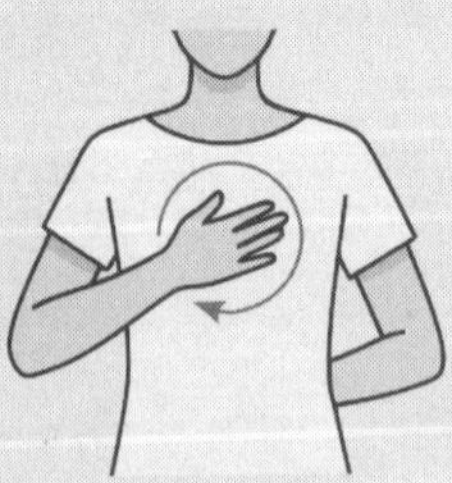

SOOTHED

If it seems right to you, hear God whispering,

As a mother comforts her child,
so will I comfort you.

ISAIAH 66:13

Allow a sense of comfort to move through your entire body—feel it deep down. Enjoy the sense of presence: your presence to your own body, and even God's presence within.

Continue with a tender "Ssshhh," perhaps adding, "I feel comforted, I feel soothed."

Soothing turns chaos into connection as calm presence quiets the storm and teaches the nervous system a new rhythm—one that lays the groundwork for character change.

STEP 2: IDENTIFY YOUR DEEP LONGINGS

As you feel more connected within, write down some deep longings of your soul. How do you want to shape your life and your character? If it might help, use the fruit of the Spirit (Galatians 5:22-23) and reflect on the shape of love in your life, the shape of joy in your life, the shape of peace in your life, etc.

As you cultivate an imagination for a life lived in love, joy, peace, and more, take the next step and feel what it would be like if you *were* living this life. Feel an embodied sense of delight, soothing, and inner connection in this state of being. (We will return to this in chapter 8.)

Stay here. Rehearse this. Come back often. This will contribute to a neural rewiring that will allow you to inhabit the life you long for.

PART 2

the maturation of character

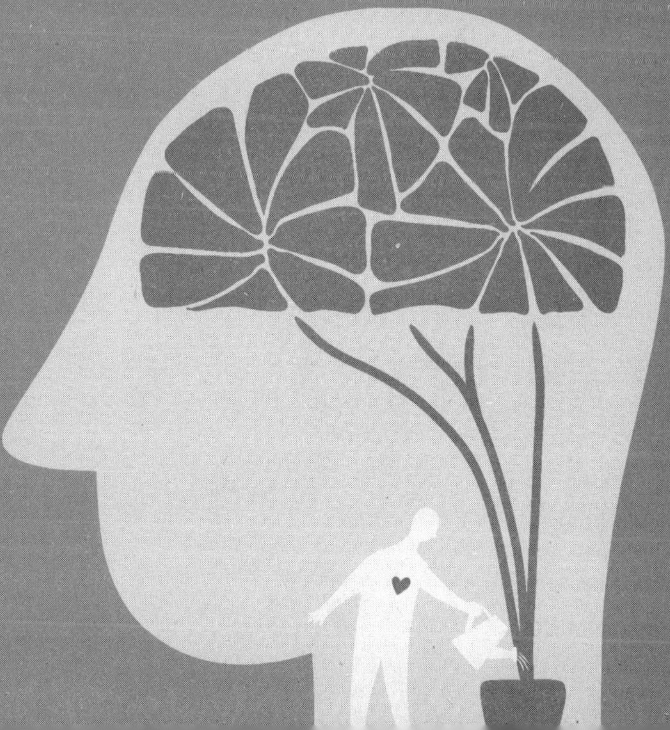

I grew up in a world where being right eclipsed being faithful.
Where factions and fences stood taller than following Jesus,
where desire was shameful,
impulse was suspect,
anxiety was sin,
and the answer was a single word—no.

I was formed in a system where correctness outweighed character,
where formulations of atonement mattered more than the fruit of love,
where doctrinal precision left discipleship gasping for air.
We debated whether our neighbor was elect
while forgetting to love them.
We honored beliefs
but ignored the world's ache.
We spoke of God's justice
but averted our eyes from injustice.
We drew lines in the sand
and called it holiness.
Certainty reigned; humility was lost.
And God?
God looked less like a loving parent
and more like an anxious warden.

I didn't know how to love myself.
I didn't know how to love the world.
I didn't know how to love God.

So I began to grow up.

Not by grasping tighter,
but by letting go.
By following Jesus
instead of fleeing heresy.
By trusting my heart's deep currents
instead of condemning its depths.
By confessing the sins not just of self,
but of systems.
By crossing the lines love demands,
rather than guarding the lines fear draws.

I'm still learning—
how to love,
how to follow,
even how to believe.
I'm dying, day by day,
to what I was told would save me
but only ever shamed me.

And I am discovering—
that Jesus' yoke is easy.
His burden, light.
Deep rest is possible
after a life of reactivity.

To grow up,
you must unlearn everything first.
You must embrace what you once exiled,
both in the world and within your own soul.

You must look up,
and see the Father's arms—open wide—
even as you're still clutching your last defense of being right.
You must let love reach your body,
especially when your body has lived locked and armored.

You must see:
All is love.
All is love.
And all will finally be resolved
in love.

CHAPTER 4

ripened

Suffering and the Slow Way of Maturity

There is no such thing as a lone wail. Every howl reverberates off the walls of God's chest and finds its way back to us, carrying his own tears with it.
COLE ARTHUR RILEY

Very truly I tell you, unless a kernel of wheat falls to the ground and dies, it remains only a single seed. But if it dies, it produces many seeds.
JOHN 12:24

My wife, Sara, once sent me on a grocery run years ago when our kids were still little. My then eight-year-old daughter Maggie came along for the ride, but she was really there for the bananas.

I scanned the pile of bananas at our local grocery store, eventually grabbing the best-looking, brightest yellow bunch I could find. And Maggie was quick to grab one just before we headed home.

I helped her start to pull back the peel, only to hear her let out a loud, "Eww" as soon as she bit into it. The banana was unripe, but I didn't know that. I couldn't tell. I didn't eat bananas.

I told Sara, "They looked great!"

"Yeah, looks can be deceiving," she responded.

She invited me to squeeze the banana, to notice that it felt harder than it should have. I learned an important lesson that day: Good looks can veil a bad banana.

When the ripening process happens as intended, fruit naturally matures, transforming from an unripe, hard, and often bitter state into something soft, sweet, and nourishing. Many fruits ripen through the release of ethylene gas, a plant hormone that signals the fruit to convert starches into sugars, producing that longed for softness and sweetness. As fruit ripens, its cell walls begin to break down, making it tender and palatable, ready to eat. The conditions are important: Fruit ripens in response to its environment—sunlight, warmth, and time are necessary. If fruit is picked too early, it may never fully ripen. If left alone too long, it may overripen and decay.

The process hinges on patient waiting.

Quite predictably, modern science has developed technology to circumvent this slow maturation process, to "force ripen" fruit with artificial gases. Fruit like bananas and tomatoes are often harvested unripe and later exposed to ethylene gas to trigger artificial ripening. It gets the job done, right? It's the reason we can eat avocados in January!

Here's the trouble—the fruit often looks mature but lacks taste and depth.

Perhaps we might call it *performative ripening*.

This is not just a story about fruit, my friends.

Avoiding Our Pain

Indeed, the temptation to appear ripened—and to appear ripened as quickly as possible—is strong. Perhaps you've found yourself captivated, like I was, by that smooth, perfectly yellow banana, deceived into thinking that it is tender, tasty, and ready to eat. I've been fooled by a few unripe bananas in my time.

Isn't this precisely what we see around us today?

- The young prodigy bursting with charisma and charm, thrust onto the stage before his character has caught up
- The polished and photogenic influencer, dispensing a wisdom clearly beyond her years
- The justice seeker, who names the pain of the world but hasn't metabolized his own
- The premature author, who got the contract because a blog post went viral
- The self-proclaimed trauma expert, who read a few books but hasn't done the work
- The overwhelmed young mother, who wasn't emotionally ready to have a child
- The anxious child, burdened with adult responsibilities at too early an age

In our chase after image, success, and efficiency, we end up circumventing long-known and time-honored pathways of ripening, pathways that invariably take us through the wilderness of suffering.

I'm reminded of the time in my first pastoral role when, after I'd offered a welcome and given announcements during the service, my senior pastor advised that I should present myself to the congregation with more energy, more enthusiasm, more gusto—to stop being so "melancholic" up there.

We'd been singing an upbeat praise song based on Psalm 42, a cheery tune led by our very talented worship band and leaders. Under the bright lights and with big smiles, we were singing words based on David's confession: "Why, my soul, are you downcast? Why so disturbed within me? Put your hope in God" (verse 5).

Beyond the sting of being called melancholic, I realized that we were singing a biblical lament as a praise song. Psalm 42 beautifully honors the heart's complexity, revealing an internal dialogue between a part of the psalmist that groans in pain and a part that longs for some kind of hope. The psalm itself is melancholic—it names suffering, grief, agony, and disorientation while grasping for relief. And it gives us permission to bring every part of ourselves to God.

Instead of fostering a journey through those deep emotions, our leadership felt it was more important to "manage the momentum" of the church experience. A popular church philosophy of the day, the idea was that the spiritual vitality of a congregation could be sustained through a carefully sequenced set of emotionally uplifting moments.

Sunday mornings were designed to be high energy and celebratory, often featuring upbeat worship and practical, inspirational messages meant to leave people "on a high." Midweek gatherings or small groups then served to recharge the soul before the next Sunday, creating a rhythm of emotional elevation.

This rhythm, the philosophy asserted, would prevent spiritual drop-off by ensuring people always had something to look forward to—another hit of energy or inspiration. In practice, what we were creating was a subtle emotional dependency on an upbeat, inspiring product—and an expectation that worship should feel a certain way. And if it didn't, chances were people would go looking elsewhere for that feeling.

You might ask: What do people do with their pain in a place like this?

We've settled for "euphoric, celebrative notions of faith that romantically pretend that life is sweetness and joy," the late biblical scholar Walter Brueggemann writes, and we've "driven the hurtful side of experience either into obscure corners of faith practice or completely out of Christian worship into various forms of psychotherapy and growth groups."[1]

Indeed, that's exactly what I saw. It was during those years that I saw how a worship experience could functionally fracture a soul. Rather than honoring the two voices in Psalm 42, this kind of worship experience unwittingly severed the soul, exiling painful parts to the shadows. If people found a safe place in other church ministries like AA meetings, the divorce care group, or with a counselor, they'd put the mask back on for Sunday mornings. I saw so many who had little idea of what to do with the pain they carried.

"The most tempting . . . is to forget [pain], to hide it, to cover it over, to pretend it never happened," said Frederick Buechner, "because it is too hard to deal with. It is too unsettling to remember." He continues:

> I think the world is always asking us to do it that way. Our families are always, in a way, . . . [saying], "Don't talk about things that cause pain. You can't trust the world with those secrets. Those are family secrets. Keep them hidden. Keep them hidden from each other. Even keep them hidden from yourself. Don't allow yourself to feel them."[2]

I have decades of stories—not least, my own—that bear witness to this internal divide. It's not an outlier; it's an epidemic. Many of our church and family systems force us to be fractured, divided within, locking away our painful experiences in the psychological dungeon.

Absent clear and intentional pathways of discipleship, formation, and what Buechner calls "the stewardship of pain," we're left without a map for the journey, without a way of processing suffering, without guides who embody the cruciform way of Jesus, without a community reflecting the breadth and depth of human experience portrayed in the psalms. We're left to wonder how it is that suffering produces perseverance, perseverance ripens character, and character grows hope. We're left to wonder how we ripen.

Four Conditions for a Sacred Ripening

The often-quoted passage about how "suffering produces perseverance; perseverance, character" wasn't written in a vacuum (Romans 5:3-4). Its context is important.

It's not *that* we suffer—it's *how* we hold and metabolize our suffering that matters.

And Paul offers some context. Transformation is possible "because God's love has been poured out into our hearts through the Holy Spirit, who has been given to us" (Romans 5:5). Or as John would say, because God first loved us (see 1 John 4:19).

Think about it this way: It's because we're safely held, known, and loved by God that we can face our suffering for the sake of character formation. It's what we know psychologically. Absent safe and connected relationship, we self-protect and disconnect, driving us further into a troubling and potentially traumatizing survival orientation. But it's within relationship—a connection orientation—that suffering can be fully digested and transformed within us.

The clearest map I found to this type of relationship showed up one Thursday afternoon at an old Borders bookstore that had become my second home. To my surprise, it wasn't psychology or Scripture that gave me the perspective I was looking for; it was the ancient initiatory traditions.

I was paging through a book by the social philosopher and family therapist Michael Gurian when I came across four core conditions for male initiation that he'd discerned—conditions that could very well apply to female initiation as well: safety, eldering, community, and a sacred story.[3]

I now see that these factors closely correspond to our early needs for attachment and authenticity. In others words, our suffering can offer us maturation, but this is not best learned under duress. It can't happen when we're stuck in a survival orientation. Our souls and bodies need space, time, relationship, and safety to metabolize fully what suffering might teach us.

Through initiatory traditions, each of us is invited on a journey meant to grow us into adulthood, filled with challenging experiences meant to test us, stretch us, and mature us. However, what we've largely lost are the surrounding conditions necessary for this transformation to take hold.

Consider each of the four core conditions for initiation:

- *Safety:* Feeling emotionally and physically secure. We need to feel safe in order to open ourselves to the vulnerability required for transformation. Without safety, self-protective instincts override the possibility of true change.
- *Eldering:* The steady presence of wise and invested mentors—women and men who see us, who've walked ahead of us, who

model maturity, and whose own scars are visible. We need these elders to journey with us through the trials that shape character.

- *Community:* A fellowship of support, challenge, and belonging. Community provides a place where we're accompanied, where we're safe enough to share ourselves (even the parts of us most others don't see), and where we're held when we do suffer.
- *A Sacred Story:* A larger meaning-making story. This allows us the broader vision to see that our sufferings aren't pointless, that life isn't hopeless, and that there is a map home.

SAFETY

Feeling emotionally and physically secure in order to open ourselves to the vulnerability required for transformation

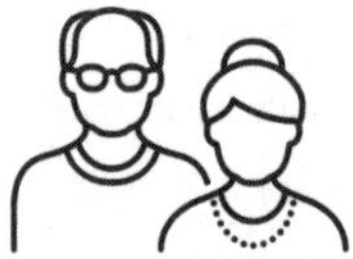

ELDERING

The steady presence of wise and invested mentors

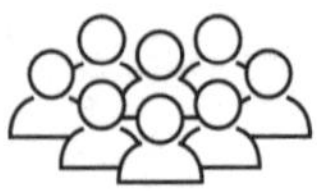

COMMUNITY

A fellowship of support, challenge, and belonging

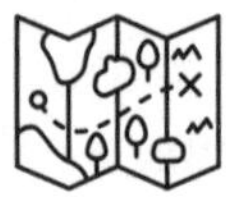

A SACRED STORY

A larger meaning-making story

Ideally, this is the kind of atmosphere the church would offer, both in its weekly and yearly liturgical rhythms and in discipleship relationships, small groups, and more. It would be astounding to see spaces where young women and men could experience meaningful passageways for their journey into adulthood.

But sadly, it's rare to find spaces like this. Many of the people I work with are sincere in their desire to follow Jesus, to live faithfully, to pray, to love—but while they've learned the "right" beliefs and are trying to do the "right" things, they find themselves adrift, wondering if the flourishing Jesus speaks of will ever find them.

This is where Denise and Matt found themselves. Both bright, driven, and ambitious, they met in college and fell in love quickly. They married in their twenties and threw themselves into building a life: careers, kids, a mortgage, church involvement—the works. He went to men's ministry events. She volunteered with a local faith-based social services agency. On the outside, everything looked admirable. But inside, something essential had been missing all along.

Neither had been initiated into the deeper realities of life—not through a rite, not through mentorship, not through the kind of soulful suffering that turns pain into wisdom. Their families had taught them to *cope*, not to *ripen*. Pain was either minimized or managed, never metabolized.

By their early forties, the character cracks were beginning to show.

Matt, successful but deeply bored at work, found himself in a quiet existential drift. He began fantasizing about escape—a cabin in the woods, a motorcycle road trip, another woman who might make him feel alive again. He couldn't name it, but he was aching for something more, something sacred, something *true*. Instead, he numbed himself with podcasts, bourbon, and an affair he swore was "just emotional."

Denise was fraying. Years of raising kids, tending a household, and managing her own career had left her brittle. Her faith, once vibrant, now felt hollow. She oscillated between rage and numbness, snapping at her kids, withdrawing from Matt. She began to wonder if this marriage—or her whole life—had been a mistake.

What neither of them could see was that they were encountering the natural *thresholds* of midlife. But they had no framework, no guide, no inner compass to help them cross through.

They lacked *safety*. As children, vulnerability had been dangerous. Both had learned to perform rather than live from their inscape, their true selves. Now, in their pain, they didn't know how to speak without attacking or retreating. Every attempt at honesty triggered shame or defensiveness. There was no safe ground for true self-disclosure—only land mines.

They lacked *eldering*. No older souls had walked them through these fires. No one said, "This is normal. This is holy ground. Let me walk with you." Without guidance, they mistook midlife disorientation for failure. They blamed each other, or themselves, rather than recognizing that their cracks might let the light in.

They lacked *community*. Their friendships were mostly surface level—pleasantries to other parents at school functions, waves to neighbors from their driveway, platitudes with their church small group. There was no shared space where their secrets could be told. So they bore their burdens in isolation, believing they were alone in their unraveling.

And even though they'd gone to church throughout their lives, Matt and Denise lacked a *sacred story*. Their understanding of life was linear: be good, work hard, succeed, stay positive. Suffering had no place in their theology. They had no sense of the cruciform, narrative arc of Scripture. It wasn't embodied within their church experience, where praise songs drowned out pain. So when the darkness came—vocational disillusionment, marital breakdown, spiritual doubt—they felt betrayed by God. No one had taught them that the soul grows through descent. That resurrection only follows crucifixion. That suffering can be sacred soil.

Models, Mentors, and Maps

I was asked to meet with a twentysomething worship pastor whose string of affairs had recently been exposed. When I asked how his career began, he paused, visibly disoriented, as if the early years had blurred together.

"I was on stage as a middle schooler as soon as I could strum a few chords," he said. "I had the voice, I guess. And people told me I looked the part . . . like a worship leader."

But when I gently asked if anyone had ever truly discipled him—walked with him, known him—he shook his head. His eyes dropped, heavy with regret. He had started cheating on the woman who would become his wife when they were still dating.

"Affairs made me feel . . . seen," he admitted quietly. "They made me feel alive."

I then had the opportunity to sit with a few of the elders and pastors at the church where the young worship pastor had served. They were clearly disappointed and surprised by the revelations. But they were just as flabbergasted when I turned the focus on them and on their church system. I asked them about the kind of church that elevates a thirteen-year-old to the stage without any intentional care, discipleship, or formation process.

"God was clearly doing something, and we didn't want to get in his way," one of them said.

It didn't take long to see that this wasn't at all about one unripened banana—a whole system that prioritized image, efficiency, and results was implicated. On the surface, they preached grace, but beneath it pulsed a quiet urgency—a drive to platform giftedness before character had time to form.

How do we steward a community of deep and safe belonging where suffering can be held and processed within a sacred story? How do we steward pathways of growth into emotional and spiritual adulthood with care and intentionality? It's a tender tension, similar to the one I carry as a parent: How do I create a safe harbor for my children while not shielding them from the very suffering that deepens the soul?

As I reflected on these questions, I began looking for models, mentors, and maps that would provide pathways of tension: places to wrestle, even suffer, for the sake of maturity. Eventually, that led me to explore ancient and non-Western initiatory traditions in my early PhD work.

And what I found stunned me: I discovered experiential initiatory rites that prized communities of deep belonging and processes of sacred suffering.

Across traditions, I discovered community rites of passage focused on nurturing belonging, forming an identity, cultivating responsibility, navigating suffering through sacred rituals, and learning surrender—priorities I didn't see in contemporary models. I found practices with echoes in the ancient Christian tradition, but these were either missing or underdeveloped in current Christian spaces.

These initiatory pathways were diverse—tracking an antelope in the wild, venturing on a Native American quest into the wilderness, even swimming in shark-infested waters or deep diving without equipment—each meant to stretch a boy through difficult circumstances, where frustration and failure would be inevitable. These distinct cultural rituals were meant to teach a boy that while he'd been the center of the story in his youth, he'd now need to discover a story much larger and durable to take into adulthood.[4] We see echoes of this in the early Christian tradition, through the catechumenate, baptismal renunciations, and even the costly witness of martyrdom, which apprenticed believers in a story shaped by the cross. Like the rites of passage in other cultures, Christian initiation marked the end of being the center of one's own narrative and the beginning of participation in a far more expansive story.

Similarly, as psychotherapist Christy Angelle Bauman shows, women's rites throughout history have often embraced processes of sacred belonging, inner transformation, descent, embodiment, and wisdom gained through life's cycles—birth, menstruation, fertility, and death.[5] Like the initiation rites of men, these, too, were intentionally stewarded by the elders and community, and they were meant to mark a path from childhood into adulthood. Here, we also see a resonance within the Christian tradition, as women like St. Teresa of Ávila, Lady Julian of Norwich, and St. Hildegard of Bingen wrote of profound spiritual initiations that came through divine encounters and intimacy, a wound of love, and transformation.

While these vital formative pathways are lacking today within Western Christian spaces, we see echoes of them in Scripture—in Israel's long desert wandering, in Jonah's three nights in a whale's belly, in Ruth's grief journey, in Mary's labor pains, in Paul's three days of blindness and three years of desert solitude—even in the wilderness temptations Jesus endured. Scripture seems to suggest that we're both held safe in God's unfathomable love *and* invited on a cruciform journey, all for the sake of our ripening.

Absent models, mentors, and maps today, we're seeing the painful consequences of a failure to maintain these pathways of initiation and maturation. Consider the stories we've seen in this book thus far. They each reveal ways in which we've lost sight of the core conditions and avenues for deep transformation. So many of the painful stories I encounter in my work are of women and men stuck in a perpetual spiritual and emotional adolescence—people who look ripe on the outside but whose souls are profoundly unripened. We often blame the individual, but we're all implicated. Our systems and spaces speak boldly of sin and grace, calling and Kingdom, and yet we've not been apprenticed in this sacred and cruciform ripening.

Together, we're invited to discern how our communities and churches can become places that foster intentional safety, eldering, community, and a sacred story. These core conditions must be embraced, not just in the abstract, but as lived and embodied realities.

Ripening into Maturity

It would be tempting at this point to offer a packaged remedy, a new spiritual formation or discipleship pathway, or a step-by-step process. But I've learned over thirty years of ministry and counseling that each story is unique. I know the sacred shape of the journey to be cruciform, but how that's embodied looks very different in each person.

And so, I've been helped by listening to and learning from the stories of women and men who've experienced this ripening. Like Viktor Frankl, a Holocaust survivor and psychiatrist, who discovered meaning in the most meaningless suffering. Or Nelson Mandela, who after twenty-seven years in prison emerged without bitterness, embodying forgiveness and leading with moral authority as he guided South Africa through reconciliation and the dismantling of apartheid.

Or Etty Hillesum, who died in a prison camp at Auschwitz at the age of twenty-nine.

Less known, Etty's is a remarkable story, captured in journals translated long after her death. In the face of encroaching terror and inevitable death from the invading Nazi forces, she had every reason to secure her defenses. Yet Etty found an unshakable inner sanctuary and profound safety through her evolving relationship with God.

She describes how she learned to turn inward, there discovering a wellspring of presence—a God who did not rescue her from suffering in the way she might have hoped, but who met her in it. This inner safety and divine companionship grounded her, ripening her under the most difficult circumstances, allowing her to walk through deep anguish without being undone by despair—even as she faced the horrors of the Holocaust.

Consider the wisdom she'd gained by her late twenties:

> And you must be able to bear your sorrow; even if it seems to crush you, you will be able to stand up again, for human beings are so strong, and your sorrow must become an integral part of yourself, part of your body and your soul, you mustn't run away from it, but bear it like an adult. Do not relieve your feelings through hatred, do not seek to be avenged on all German mothers, for they, too, sorrow at this very moment for their slain and murdered sons. Give your sorrow all the space and shelter in yourself that is its due, for if everyone bears his grief honestly and courageously, the sorrow that now fills the world will abate. But if you do not

> clear a decent shelter for your sorrow, and instead reserve most of the space inside you for hatred and thoughts of revenge—from which new sorrows will be born for others—then sorrow will never cease in this world and will multiply. And if you have given sorrow the space its gentle origins demand, then you may truly say: life is beautiful and so rich. So beautiful and so rich that it makes you want to believe in God.[6]

Etty's wisdom was not gained in a sterile, suffering-proof space. Rather, it was unearthed in the midst of the terrifying inevitability of death. What shaped her?

She experienced the mentorship and counsel of wise elders. She experienced community in her friendships, such as with Maria Tuinzing, to whom she entrusted her diaries before leaving Amsterdam for good. She left to serve people being held at the Westerbork Transit Camp, a stopover for those Dutch Jews who were destined to be sent to Auschwitz. About a year later, she herself was interned at Westerbork, along with her parents and brother. She felt solidarity with her co-sufferers, both there and at Auschwitz, where she and her family were eventually sent. Finally, she experienced a sacred story by recognizing that union with God was her deepest reality, not least through her immersion in the writings of Fyodor Dostoevsky, Rainer Maria Rilke, and St. Augustine. In all of this, she discovered a remarkable safety, writing, "There is a really deep well inside me. And in it dwells God. Sometimes I am there, too." A year later, she wrote again about the need to focus on him: "And that is all we can manage these days and also all that really matters: that we safeguard that little piece of You, God, in ourselves."[7]

Etty's story is compelling, as are the stories of Nelson Mandela, Victor Frankl, and many others. But perhaps you can think of someone you know whose life reveals this transformative pattern.

I think of my friend Bruce, who passed away a few years back after a long battle with several simultaneous life-threatening conditions. Bruce retired after a long career as a math professor, often spending hours in silence and solitude, experiencing that spacious inner realm that Etty must have known. I was his pastor, twenty years younger than him, and he'd frequently visit me on Thursdays at the Borders bookstore, emerging from the silence, his eyes still heavy with stillness.

I often asked Bruce how it was to know that death was on the doorstep, and sometimes through tears he told me how loved and held he felt by God. I knew he spent long nights before the Lord, usually in great pain, his laments rising to the heavens, trusting that God was big and safe enough to hold them. Amidst my youthful reactivity, I wondered how he could be so steady and sure, even as death crept in.

We need these stories of sacred suffering. They offer us a picture of gradual ripening, even if what we crave is a quick, surefire program for spiritual growth. But while there isn't a universal guide to ripening, I'm inspired by those who are creating contemporary pathways to steward seasons of early ripening, midlife transition, suffering, dark nights of the soul, doubt, injustice, and more.

For example, my colleagues and I offer five-day therapeutic intensives. Other groups host story work retreats,[8] structured journeys through the Ignatian exercises, walking pilgrimages along Europe's Camino de Santiago, soul care cohorts, and spiritual direction training.[9]

And while I'm not as equipped to write about them, churches and Christian spaces within the Black, Hispanic, and Asian communities engage suffering through faith and justice cohorts, as well as testimony, lament liturgies, song, and even public protest.[10] Musicians also gather to put words to matters of soul often ignored in worship spaces.[11]

These offerings and practices are not all explicitly initiatory, but they can serve that function in the absence of more substantial communal pathways. Each of these experiences is an invitation into something larger, where safety, community, eldering, and sacred story are held.

I look back at my life of faith and see now that, while I was trained to think the right thoughts and do the right things, I experienced no apprenticeship in suffering—no mentors to walk alongside me, no community practiced in holding pain. I thought my tears were signals of failure, something to apologize for, not signs of my ripening.

In *This Here Flesh*, Cole Arthur Riley writes, "Every howl reverberates off the walls of God's chest and finds its way back to us, carrying his own tears with it."[12] And because of this, we can trust that our tears fall like rain into the soil of the soul, softening what was hard, nourishing hidden roots, and making possible the slow, sacred ripening of character.

And so, dear friends,

May you find the safety that softens your defenses—
the kind of presence that lets your soul breathe
so the hard and hidden places might begin to open.

May you be met by wise elders—
those scarred by life, yet soft of heart,
who walk with you not to fix or hurry you,
but to hold space for your becoming.

May you discover soul companions
who see beneath the surface,
who call forth your truest self,
and create a circle of belonging
where honesty isn't punished,
and suffering is never carried alone.

May you be rooted in a sacred story—
not of perfection, but of transformation—
a story where descent is holy,
where the seed must fall and die,
where sorrow is the soil of character.

And may you trust:
what is ripening in you—
slowly, quietly,
even through suffering—
is good,
is needed,
and will bear fruit in its time.

RESOURCES

- Christy Angelle Bauman, *Her Rites: A Sacred Journey for the Mind, Body, and Soul*
- Michael J. Gorman, *Inhabiting the Cruciform God: Kenosis, Justification, and Theosis in Paul's Narrative Soteriology*
- Matthew Kaemingk and Kathryn Roelofs, *Leading Worship for Workers: How to Design Liturgies for All of Life*
- Alexander Schmemann, *For the Life of the World: Sacraments and Orthodoxy*
- John Swinton, *Raging with Compassion: Pastoral Responses to the Problem of Evil*

REFLECTION

1. Where do you notice "performative ripening" in your own life? In what roles or relationships do you feel pressure to *look* mature, even when your inner world feels unready or unfinished?
2. How has your church or family taught you to handle pain? Were you encouraged to name and feel it—or to hide, minimize, spiritualize, or manage it away?
3. Consider Gurian's four conditions for sacred ripening: safety, eldering, community, and a sacred story (see pages 103-104). Which of these have you tasted in your own life, and which have felt most absent? Can you name particular elders or guides who have helped walk you through these stages?
4. In your experience, what is the context for character transformation? What stages does it entail? For instance, did your family or expanded circle provide some version of an initiation or a mentorship to guide you into maturity? In what ways does your church or another group you belong to provide such a space?

5. How do you respond to the idea that "the soul grows through descent" (page 107)? Does this feel hopeful, threatening, confusing, or clarifying? Why?

6. As you imagine your own initiation into deeper adulthood or maturity, what might it need to include right now—what truth to face, what grief to honor, what risk to take, what support to seek?

PRACTICE

Cultivating Ripening for the Sake of Character Change

Naming the Story That Shaped Your Understanding of Suffering

Set aside ten to fifteen minutes with a journal.

STEP 1: IDENTIFY THE STORY YOU INHERITED

Write about the messages—explicit or implicit—you received about suffering from your family, church, culture, or early relationships. You might consider the following:

- What were you taught to do with your pain?
- Was suffering something to hide? Endure? Ignore? "Get over"?
- Were certain emotions off-limits?
- What stories (biblical or not) were used to frame hardship?
- Did anyone model honest lament, or was that discouraged?

STEP 2: NOTICE HOW THIS STORY LIVES IN YOU TODAY

Describe how this inherited story still shapes your reactions:

- How do you tend to respond when you're hurting?
- What parts of you emerge—parts that are protective, parts that perform, parts that avoid, parts that get angry?

- What internal scripts do you still hear (e.g., "be strong"; "don't burden others"; "just trust God")?

STEP 3: NAME THE CONSEQUENCES

Gently notice how this story has helped you survive, but also how it may have limited your ability to ripen.

- Write without judgment. Just witness.

Re-Storying Your Life Within a Sacred Narrative

This practice is a way of embodying a new, larger story—one that honors suffering, holds it in love, and opens the possibility of transformation.

Choose whichever medium feels right: reflective or poetic writing, drawing, praying, collaging, moving, or following a guided imaginative exercise.

STEP 1: BEGIN WITH BREATH

Let your breath slow. Imagine yourself held in God's compassionate presence—like a seed held in soil.

STEP 2: INVITE A PAINFUL PART OF YOU FORWARD

Picture the part of you that still carries hurt, disappointment, exhaustion, or regret. Not the whole story—just a part.

Let this part of you be seen. Offer it gentle acknowledgment: *You've carried so much. Thank you.*

STEP 3: PLACE THIS PART WITHIN THE LARGER SACRED STORY

Now imagine this part of you standing in the landscape of a sacred text or mythic moment. You may want to revisit Scripture for images of sacred suffering:

- in the wilderness with Israel
- in the whale's belly with Jonah, waiting for light

- in Mary's labor pains
- in Jesus' desert temptation
- with Ruth in her grief
- in Paul's blindness
- in a psalm of lament
- with Jesus in his final hours
- at the tomb before dawn

As an alternative, you could picture this part of you alongside Etty Hillesum, Nelson Mandela, or someone in your own life who has suffered well.

Let this tender part of you see where it belongs—not alone, but within a lineage of sacred suffering.

STEP 4: WRITE OR CREATE FROM THIS NEW PERSPECTIVE

Ask:

- What does this place reveal?
- What does the sacred story say to your suffering part?
- How does it shift the meaning of what you've endured?
- What becomes possible in this larger frame?

Then express it:

Write a first-person monologue from your suffering part.

Create a poem.

Sketch a scene.

Write a letter from God or from your wiser, older self to this part that carries a burden.

Make a collage of images that symbolize descent and rising.

Let the new story take shape in texture, color, language, or movement.

STEP 5: IDENTIFY THE NEW TRUTH EMERGING

Finish with one sentence that captures the heart of your re-storied narrative. Something like

> My suffering is not proof of abandonment but an invitation to ripening.
>
> This descent is part of my initiation into a truer self.
>
> I am held in a larger story even when I do not feel held.
>
> This pain is not the end of the story.
>
> God was and is with me in my most painful moments.
>
> Slowly, I am ripening.

Write your sentence somewhere visible—a small reminder of your maturing.

CHAPTER 5

reintegrated

Cultivating Integrity as Wholeheartedness (Not Moralism)

You can resolve to live your life with integrity. Let your credo be this: Let the lie come into the world, let it even triumph. But not through me.
ALEKSANDR SOLZHENITSYN

Everything exposed by the light becomes visible—and everything that is illuminated becomes a light.
EPHESIANS 5:13

Jen had finally made it.

She'd long been the best student in her classes—disciplined, thoughtful, dependable. She pushed hard through her PhD, learning to live on deadlines and determination, telling herself she could rest later. When she landed a faculty position, it felt like arrival: a full teaching load, eager students, collegial affirmation. She looked, by all accounts, like someone who had done everything right.

But behind the outer competence, Jen was beginning to crack.

Her schedule was relentless. Her inbox never emptied. She carried high expectations, many of them her own. And she met them by ignoring the quiet signals of fatigue. She told herself this was normal, the cost of meaningful work.

Jen had always wanted to be helpful. Raised in a family where worth was tethered to achievement and reliability, she learned early to earn belonging by excelling and by saying yes. Over time, that *yes* became reflexive, hollowed of desire, aimed to please. The anxious, angry, and exhausted parts of her had no place in the life she'd built, so she kept them buried.

Until they surfaced.

The panic attack came in the middle of an ordinary afternoon. Her heart raced. Her breath shortened. The room felt unreal. She closed her office door and slid to the floor, frightened.

That evening, Jen made a call she'd never allowed herself to make. She let someone see the whole of her—overwhelm and all.

That courageous call did not mark her failure. It marked the beginning of her reintegration.

Out of Alignment

As we've seen, when we are dis-integrated—fragmented from our unique inscape and true selves—we operate from isolated parts rather than a unified whole. We wear masks, even spiritual-looking ones. Like Adam and Eve after grasping the fruit, we hide behind fig leaves, self-protective and projecting whatever part we believe will help us manage the moment.

As Jen discovered, however, living a dis-integrated life comes at a cost. The parts of us we bury don't stay silent—they seep out, sabotage, and scapegoat. In time, we feel divided within—as if we're living a contradiction. The apostle Paul named the internal dynamic succinctly and practically when he wrote, "I do not understand what I do. For what I want to do I do not do, but what I hate I do" (Romans 7:15).

What results is performance rather than presence: justice-seeking that masks a need to be seen as righteous, caretaking that disguises a fear of rejection, spiritual maturity that projects certainty while hiding doubt, even self-awareness that curates a faux vulnerability without true transformation. Such actions often perpetuate confusion, manipulation, or control. When this happens, our unacknowledged fragmentation becomes a burden others are forced to carry—in our parenting, our leadership, and our friendships.

Even when these performative actions appear righteous, virtuous, or composed on the surface, they lack *integrity*, a coherent and integrated true self, grounded in love. And when it comes to true character, the root of the actions makes all the difference.

I often hear people say, "We need more integrity in our leaders." And I agree. But I wonder: Are we all operating from the same definition of integrity? Too often the sentiment behind this statement is a desire—even an expectation—of moral purity. And too often, what we call character is little more than a curated or idealized self—a persona shaped to fit external expectations.

Integrity, however, is not about moral perfection; it's about wholeness—a life lived in integration rather than fragmentation. The word shares its root with *integer*, meaning "whole" or "undivided." This vision of integrity is less about spotless performance and more about the courageous work of becoming internally aligned.[1]

It's an important distinction to highlight as we journey toward a maturing character: Integrity means allowing our outer life to echo our inner life, *not* by eliminating our shadows but by integrating them so that what once ruled us from the dark is transformed in the light and we dare to live as our whole, complete selves.

The Ancient Work of an Aligned Heart

These ideas are not new, nor are they pithy psychological takes lacking the depth of biblical and theological substance.

This language resonates with something ancient—the soul's longing for oneness, for union, even as we're tempted to grasp for what we think will satisfy us. As early as the fourth century, St. Augustine wrote, "You are torn apart by these many loves, restless everywhere and nowhere at peace. Gather yourself together into your real self. If anything outside you has been giving you joy, ask who is its maker."[2]

Long before Carl Jung mapped the psyche in psychological terms or trauma therapists named the realities of fragmentation and integration, the desert fathers and mothers described a strikingly similar inner landscape. For these early Christian sages, the human heart was a battleground of conflicting desires and disordered attachments—like anger, pride, gluttony, vainglory. If left unexamined, these passions, temptations, and burdensome thoughts shape us from the depths, sabotaging our life with God and others by fragmenting our attention and distorting our loves. "If you are not aware of the thoughts that assail you," the Christian monk Evagrius Ponticus wrote in the fourth century, "you will not be able to perceive the things that happen to you."[3]

Centuries later, the psychologist Carl Jung would name this the "shadow"—the unconscious part of ourselves that contains the thoughts, emotions, and desires we reject, repress, or deny, often because they conflict with our ideal self-image. Today, we might notice a part of ourselves we don't like and proclaim, "I hate that about myself!" Or "I wish I could get rid of that part of me!" But both ancient and contemporary wisdom call not for suppression or eradication but for spiritual differentiation—seeing what is motivated by love, and what is not.

In our day, author and educator Parker Palmer provides a framework to help us trace the stories of our inner divisions:

> We arrive in this world with birthright gifts—then we spend the first half of our lives abandoning them or letting others disabuse us of them. As young people, we are surrounded by expectations that may have little to do with who we really are, expectations held by people who are not trying to discern our selfhood but to fit us into slots. In families, schools, workplaces, and religious communities, we are trained away from true self toward images of acceptability; under social pressures like racism and sexism our original shape is deformed beyond recognition; and we ourselves, driven by fear, too often betray true self to gain the approval of others. We are disabused of original giftedness in the first half of our lives. Then—if we are awake, aware, and able to admit our loss—we spend the second half trying to recover and reclaim the gift we once possessed.[4]

Palmer's wisdom is helpful in our journey toward becoming ourselves. So is this insight from the author and civil rights pioneer James Baldwin: "Not everything that is faced can be changed; but nothing can be changed until it is faced."[5] And that long look in the mirror is painful.

Becoming Whole

This willingness to sit with our discomfort is where the work of integration begins. It's here where integrity begins—where we give up the impossible burden of perfecting ourselves, managing our image, or performing our virtue.

Sitting with discomfort can be painful though. Jen worked hard to rid herself of her lifelong distress, rooted early in life when she felt like a burden, a failure, inadequate. Many of us find ways to circumvent our dis-ease. We scroll to soothe. We drink to disconnect. We overwork to avoid. You won't see bumper stickers and T-shirts that say "Sit with discomfort," but you will see some that read "Hustle" or "Good Vibes Only."

Consider this: We often suffer not because of our mistakes but because of our attempts at perfection. My mom put a magnet on our refrigerator that haunted me for years: "Be perfect as your Father in heaven is perfect" (Matthew 5:48, GW). I learned to manage an image of moral uprightness, relegating the dark side of myself to the shadows. Sadly, my character was shaped in those days around an absence of integrity, as I was living a divided life—all in a convoluted attempt to live an upright life!

When we read the words of Jesus in Matthew, "Be perfect" (*teleios* in Greek), we're often misled by bad translation. *Teleios* is better translated "mature" or "whole."[6] It expresses not how we should properly behave, but who we can become. *Teleios* speaks of a soul gathered from its fragments, of fear no longer driving the story, of desire purified by surrender, of strength softened by compassion. And as we've seen, the hope is that we can become ourselves—integrated, whole, one.

The thirteenth-century German mystic Mechthild of Magdeburg wrote, "The noblest joy of the senses, the holiest peace of the heart, and the greatest delight in doing come from keeping one's integrity in all that one does."[7] Søren Kierkegaard echoes this six centuries later, writing, "Purity of heart is to will one thing."[8]

This is the life of integrity—a life of inner alignment, with each and every scattered part brought compassionately into the light, allowing us to be a light to others. Because becoming whole is not about perfection but about illumination and integration.

Expanding on his vision of maturation, Paul reminds us that "everything exposed by the light becomes visible—and everything that is illuminated becomes a light" (Ephesians 5:13).

Jen's panic attack would jump-start her own journey, awakening a need for therapeutic care, but she was anxious. She'd lived an ordered life and was worried therapy might "open up a can of worms" that she'd not be able to contain. The work that followed, however, felt less chaotic and out of control than she'd imagined, as she was invited to slowly turn her gaze toward parts of herself that she had spent a lifetime outrunning.

She discovered these inner parts and began to name them: an overfunctioning achiever who believed rest was weakness; a vigilant analyst scanning for disapproval; an angry little girl within who had never felt safe enough to speak; a sad little one who never felt like she was enough. Instead of silencing them, she grew curious. What were they protecting? What did they fear would happen if she said no? How were they burdened?

Jen slowed down. She began to sense discomfort and stay with it. She practiced noticing the tightening in her chest before agreeing to one more request. She experimented with limits—small noes that felt both terrifying and freeing. She grieved the childhood equation that fused love with performance. She began distinguishing between her true desires and the reflex to please.

The more she stayed with her distress, the more it lost its power. Anxious parts calmed. Scrupulosity waned. Sadness didn't devour her but softened her. Colleagues noticed that she was smiling more.

Integration did not mean abandoning ambition or dulling her gifts. It meant gathering the fragmented pieces of herself into a more honest whole. It meant learning to abide rather than strive, to work from a steadier center rather than from an anxious edge. Slowly, her yeses became more rooted—less compulsive, more chosen. And as her inner life grew more aligned, the panic loosened its grip.

Wholeness begins when we dare to let the light of truth reach the parts of us we've kept hidden—our wounds, our shame, our contradictions—all for the sake of integrity, or wholeness of heart. It means turning toward, not away from, the internal divisions we've learned to conceal. And that's what Jen did. In fact, before this, she'd spent so much time outside herself, focused on her research and her students, that she was surprised by how good it felt to curate a greater sense of peace and oneness within. And she was sure that she'd experienced a new sense of communion with God through it.

In God's economy, this inward gaze is never for condemnation; it's for transformation. What we bring into the light doesn't just become visible; it becomes light itself—transfigured, healed, and capable of offering light to others.

Psalm 51 emerges from one of the most devastating moments of moral failure in King David's life. There is no way to sugarcoat it—his actions included abuse of power, betrayal, concealment, and a calculated murder plot following his exploitation of Bathsheba, all under the guise of royal power and privilege. When the prophet Nathan shines a light on David (see 2 Samuel 12), his defenses finally break, and he turns inward—not just in remorse, but in search of reintegration. His cry, "What you're after is truth from the inside out. Enter me, then; conceive a new, true life" (Psalm 51:6, MSG), reveals a man reckoning with the deep fracture between who he had become and who he was meant to be.

After his collapse, David longed not just for pardon, but for this kind of purity of heart: "Create in me a pure [טָהוֹר or *tahor* in Hebrew] heart, O God, and renew a steadfast spirit within me" (Psalm 51:10, NIV). He seeks a pure heart, an undivided heart, a heart that wills one thing, as Kierkegaard wrote. In that cry, we glimpse not just remorse but the beginning of reintegration—a man no longer managing appearances, but yielding to the inner work of becoming whole, honest, and undivided before God. This was the beginning of the inner work, mind you, not the completion of it.

Perhaps Jesus had this story in mind when he offered the Beatitude, "Blessed are the pure [*katharos*] in heart, for they will see God" (Matthew 5:8). Notice the strong semantic connection between the words of David and Jesus. The Greek word *katharos* points to something whole, unmixed, and sincere.[9] In a world full of performative piety, Jesus blesses those who bring their full selves into the light—not just their strengths, but their shadows. To be pure in heart is not to be flawless, but to be integrated—to let the light shine into every room of the soul, until even what was hidden becomes whole. The entire vision of the beatitudes is for the sake of becoming salt and light to the world (Matthew 5:13-16).

But all of this doesn't happen in an instant. The biblical vision isn't hinting at an Instagram apology and a comeback tour. It doesn't suggest a recipe or a set of techniques to achieve one's best life in as little time as possible. As Scripture suggests, sometimes it takes a long wilderness journey to find our way home.

The Slow Rebuild

"How long will it take?" may be the question I hear the most as I work with Christian leaders embarking on a journey of character transformation. Most realize soon enough that the work of heart excavation and re-formation is measured not in minutes and days but in years and decades. It's not simply about taking a month away as a short breather from leadership. It is about reckoning with the depth of division within. It's not simply about forgiving and forgetting. It's tough to forgive others if we've not been reconciled internally ourselves.

One pastor told me several years into the work, "I preached that—but I never thought it applied to me." Another common sentiment.

And so we begin to see just how long it takes to become whole.

When we've named the masks, the shame, the buried ache, the false selves we constructed to cope or belong, when we start to experience the slow undoing of old survival strategies and the tender reawakening of what lies beneath, we begin to discern the depth of the work—and the duration of it, as well. When we're able to stay with the shame long enough for it to soften in the light of mercy, we begin to discover that what once felt unbearable is not the end of us.

We may sense that the very strategies that once served us become the hardest to release because they shaped, not just how others saw us, but how we came to see ourselves. We recognize that shedding them means facing grief, both for what hurt us and for what we might lose by letting go. And we see the pain we've caused others—through our failures and through the protective performances that kept us from being fully present, honest, and available.

This, too, is part of the reckoning.

Jen discovered that just as it had taken years for her to construct a life of order and perfection, so it would take years to cultivate the internal safety she needed for the wholeness she longed for. After several years of doing this work, she said to me, "A deep sense of rest is beginning to be my default mode. And it's so freeing. I didn't realize just how tightly I was gripping the wheel for so long—and how that didn't just impact me, but my friends and colleagues too."

To become whole is not only to reclaim what's been lost within us, but to acknowledge the impact we've had beyond ourselves. It is a humbling path, marked by both sorrow and reparation. But it is the only path that leads us home to ourselves and to one another.

This is the holy ache of transformation: to slowly unlearn what once kept us safely self-protected, and to risk becoming someone truer, freer, and more deeply alive.

What parts of you need light to bring about reconciliation and redemption within? What hidden places need to emerge from the shadows so that you can be transformed? And what kind of journey are you willing to go on to become *wholly* yourself?

And so, dear friends,

May you find the courage to lay down your mask—
not in shame, but in trust—
trust that your truest self is already beloved,
even when unpolished, uncertain, or undone.

May you greet the anxious parts that once protected you—
not with contempt,
but with gratitude for how they helped you survive,
and compassion as you learn to bless and unburden them.

May the grief you carry be honored, not rushed—
the grief for what hurt you,
and the grief for how you've hurt others—
so that you might live more honestly and whole.

May you be met by companions of integrity—
those who have faced their own shadows
and now walk with humility,
offering you a space where nothing needs to be hidden.

May you come to see that becoming whole
is not about perfection,
but about light—
light that reveals, light that heals,
light that slowly matures you into a person of integrity.

And may you trust
that this lifelong work of unmasking and reintegration
is not only good and necessary,
but sacred—a return to the self
you were always meant to be.

RESOURCES

- Chuck DeGroat, *Wholeheartedness: Busyness, Exhaustion, and Healing the Divided Self*
- Molly LaCroix, *Journey to Shalom: Finding Healing, Wholeness, and Freedom in Sacred Stories*
- Elizabeth O'Connor, *Our Many Selves: A Handbook for Self-Discovery*
- Parker J. Palmer, *A Hidden Wholeness: The Journey Toward an Undivided Life*

REFLECTION

1. Where do you feel most divided between your "outer" life and your "inner" life—those places where what others see and what you actually experience don't match?

2. What masks do you wear most often (competent, caring, unbothered, spiritual, strong, etc.)? What vulnerable parts of you are those masks trying to protect?
3. How has inner division cost you in some way—whether personally in shame, guilt, even exhaustion, or more relationally, in conflict or rupture?
4. If integrity is becoming whole rather than becoming perfect, what one small step could you take this week to bring a hidden part of your story into the light—with God and with a safe, trusted person?

PRACTICE

Cultivating Reintegration for the Sake of Character Change

The fourth-century desert father Evagrius Ponticus taught people how to disentangle themselves from harmful self-protective strategies. He encouraged discernment—the prayerful naming, tending, and transformation of these forces through spiritual practices—as a means to cultivate inner attunement and loving action.

This discernment exercise is designed to help you identify and illuminate a part of yourself that you might not be aware of, one you might have even relegated to the shadows, but that is keeping you from wholeness. You might frame this as a fifteen- to twenty-minute practice, once a week.

STEP 1: SETTLE AND INVITE

Sit quietly. Take a few slow breaths. Pray something like this: "Create in me a whole heart, O God, and renew a right spirit within me" (see Psalm 51:10).

STEP 2: RECALL A MOMENT OF PERFORMANCE

Let your mind wander back over the last day or week. Choose one moment when you felt you were *performing* rather than being fully *present*—at work, on social media, in a conversation, at church.

Ask yourself,

- *What did I want others to see or believe about me in that moment?*
- *What was I afraid they might see instead?*

STEP 3: MEET THE PART OF YOU IN THE SHADOWS

Gently notice the part of you that was performing. It won't feel quite like you when you're at rest—it will feel a bit more anxious, alert, vigilant. Notice this aspect of it. Notice whatever sensations in your body accompany this part of you (a tight chest, a clenched jaw, shallow breath).

Ask that part (you can even write this out),

- What is your role?
- What are you trying to protect me from?
- What do you fear might happen to me if you didn't do your job?
- When did you first have to carry this burden?

Instead of scolding, offer kindness: *Thank you for how you've tried to protect me. You don't have to do this alone anymore.*

STEP 4: BRING THE MOMENT INTO THE LIGHT

Now imagine that moment, and that part of you, held in God's gaze and held in your gaze—no flinching, no turning away.

Pray,

- What truth do you want to speak to this part of me?
- What do I need to confess about how my hiding or defensiveness has affected others?

If needed, name any concrete harm or distance your performance created. Receive forgiveness; ask for courage to seek repair where appropriate.

STEP 5: ACT IN A NEW, INTEGRATED WAY

Ask one final question: *What is one small, specific action I can take this week that is more aligned with my true self than with my old mask?*

Examples:

telling a trusted friend the truth about your tendency to perform

saying no where you'd usually overfunction

apologizing for your negative impact on others

breathing more deeply and intentionally when prompted to perform

resting instead of pushing through

STEP 6: REST IN YOUR TRUE SELF

See what it's like to experience inner separation and differentiation when you notice that parts of you are taking over, at times, and when you are able to retune to your true self. Notice how your breathing changes when you are rested and secure, when you feel at home in yourself. Stay with this feeling long enough to breed familiarity and comfort here.

Then, spent a bit of time with Galatians 5:22-23 asking, "How might the fruits of the Spirit grow from this soil of security?"

Close with a simple blessing, perhaps, "Create in me a whole heart, O God. Bring my scattered parts into your light, and teach me to live from who I truly am in you."

You've been told the lie
(though not in so many words)
that if you don't shine
you'll disappear.
That you won't be seen
if you're not on.
That digital space is crowded
and the algorithms demand your sacrifice.
Feed the glow, they say.
Curate brilliance
(even if you don't have it in you).
The digital egosphere requires its offering.
So you polish your moments
(and trim the ragged edges),
filter the light until it flatters,
until you are palatable enough to trend.
Yet in the quiet
when the screen dims
and the crowd scrolls past,
you feel the hollowing.
What good is being seen
if I am no longer here?
What worth is relevance
if it costs me presence?

I want you to step back—
let the glow fade
let the silence swell
until you remember the shape of your own soul.
To shine, not for them,
but because
the light within
is enough.

CHAPTER 6

reoriented

Mapping the Stages of a Transformative Journey

In the beginning I was so young and such a stranger to myself I hardly existed. I had to go out into the world and see it and hear it and react to it, before I knew at all who I was, what I was, what I wanted to be.
MARY OLIVER

He who began a good work in you will carry it on to completion until the day of Christ Jesus.
PHILIPPIANS 1:6

"I don't feel like I'll ever get it right," Liz said, her face in her hands as she sat over coffee with her mentor, Pat.

Liz was a mom of three children under the age of five. Before her first was born, she had been active in her church, sensing her faith maturing through Bible studies and small groups. But this season seemed to upend that growth. She'd hit a wall, and it felt like failure, not faithfulness.

Her mentor pulled a paper napkin toward her, drawing a big *U* on it.

"Here's your map," she said.

Liz's hands dropped from her face, and she looked up with hope, saying, "I love maps!" But when she saw it, she sighed. "That's it?"

"Well, that's part of it, Liz," Pat said. "You were here," she said, pointing to the top left part of the U-curve. "And now you're here," she said, pointing to the bottom.

"It's the wilderness," Pat said. "It's the valley. And the truth is, it's not just people going through hard times who end up in valleys. Faithful people like you end up here too. We all do."

Why Maps Matter

Like Liz, we all find it challenging at times to know where we are in our quest to become who we were created to be. And often, we hit a wall along the way. If this is where you are, you're not alone.

"You've got yourself stuck in a moment / And now you can't get out of it," Bono—the lead singer of U2—cries out.[1] He captures with lyrical urgency the human experience of unresolved pain, where developmental wounds and spiritual paralysis converge, leaving the soul suspended between where we are and what we long for. Sometimes I wish it would be as easy as opening an app on my phone and following a map of the journey home.

"Christian faith is about life, and life involves unfolding process, growth to maturity and arrival at the appointed destination," writes the late theologian Bruce Demarest. "Some unwisely launch the journey without a roadmap or plan, and so wander aimlessly and suffer needlessly."[2]

The truth is, we'll inevitably get lost. And we desperately need maps, not least maps of these unfolding seasons—or stages—of a ripening and maturing life. Scripture itself, from beginning to end, speaks of seasons. Trees yield fruit in season, wisdom grows with age, and even the soul moves in cycles of pruning and renewal.[3]

The apostle Paul, as we've seen, names a journey of spiritual maturation that moves from infancy to adulthood: "until we all reach unity in the faith . . . and become mature, attaining to the whole measure of the fullness of Christ" (Ephesians 4:13).

Jesus himself speaks of losing life in order to find it (Matthew 16:25)—a process of learning to die to our pseudo-attachments, which opens the door to deeper attachment to and union with God. And he speaks about the first and second halves of life with Peter, saying, "Very truly I tell you, when you were younger you dressed yourself and went where you wanted; but when you are old you will stretch out your hands, and someone else will dress you and lead you where you do not want to go" (John 21:18).

These aren't just theological abstractions; they describe an unfolding process from disconnection to connection, from fragmentation to wholeness, from control to surrender, from alienation to union with God.

In your own life, you've likely found a helpful map or two along the way. If you've ever taken a developmental psychology class or thumbed through a book on parenting, you've probably come across maps of childhood growth. I recall a book we bought after our daughter Emma was born, charting what we should expect at key growth moments. A smile in the first six to eight weeks, a first word in the first ten to twelve months, a first "No!" around two years old. I recall Emma's first "No!" and many more after that!

From the earliest moments of bonding and trust to the slow discovery of identity and the stirrings of moral reasoning, childhood and adolescence trace paths that form the foundation for empathy, resilience, responsibility, and integrity. And if you've spent much time around kids of different ages, you've likely noticed it firsthand: Each stage carries its own set of wonders and challenges, its own unique tasks that quietly shape who we become.

The twentieth-century developmental psychologist Erik Erikson pictured these stages as thresholds, each one asking us to navigate a core tension before we can move forward. When we meet these challenges well, he suggested, we carry forward a deeper strength and a more integrated sense of self—better equipped to face what lies ahead with courage and integrity.[4] This is the integrative work we learned about in the previous chapter, but normalized through the unfolding stages of life.

What if this same sentiment applied to our spiritual lives? And what if there were maps with distinct thresholds of growth and resources to navigate them?

In fact, there are.

I first discovered this in the work of Dr. James Fowler. A theologian and human development expert, Fowler proposed a framework for understanding how faith unfolds in stages that mirror our maturation process. Just as Erikson understood that we begin moving through developmental stages from birth, Fowler recognized that faith is not a fixed posture but a dynamic process. It develops through predictable phases—from the curious trust of childhood to the growing convictions of adolescence and eventually to the hard-won, reflective faith of adulthood.

Along the way, Fowler argues, challenges such as doubt, disillusionment, or spiritual discouragement often emerge—not as *threats* to faith that must be relegated to the shadows but as *necessary disruptions* that invite deeper integration. It is through wrestling with these tensions, he says, that faith matures, shaping not only what we believe but who we become.[5] Remember that it's not what we avoid that grows us; it is what we experience and integrate that has the capacity to mature us.

Character formation, then, is not separate from human development but deeply embedded within it.

The Long and Winding Way

Perhaps you've experienced what poet Mary Oliver names:

I climb. I backtrack.
I float.
I ramble my way home.[6]

With Pat's help, Liz began to discover that the way was winding. She recognized that backtracking wasn't a sign of faithlessness and that hitting a wall wasn't failure; instead, they were an inevitable part of a faithful journey. Strangely, she'd never been offered a map before. But there were plenty to be found.

For centuries, Christians have offered trail markers along a well-worn path designed to help us find our way. In the second century, the bishop and theologian St. Irenaeus wrote, "The Creator is always the same, but those who are created must pass from a beginning and through a middle course, a growth, and progression. It is for this progress and increase that God has formed them."[7] A beginning journey leads to a midlife passage, opening us to a further journey toward God, he says.

This threefold process of orientation, disorientation, and reorientation is echoed in Scripture—and particularly in the Psalms—according to the late Old Testament theologian Walter Brueggemann.[8] Human life tends to follow a familiar path: orientation, when life holds together; disorientation, when we lose our footing; and reorientation, when we discover that the descent itself has reshaped us and opened us to a deeper gratitude and trust in God.[9]

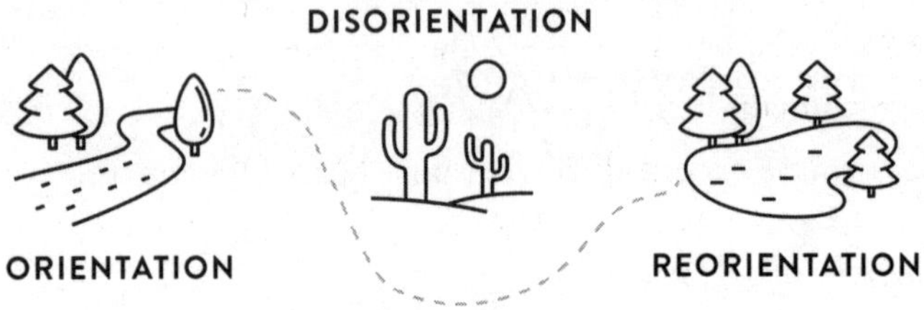

Throughout Christian history, others have developed similar maps. Some add more turns or describe the journey of faith from a different perspective, but all have the similar trajectory of orientation, disorientation, reorientation.[10] These early maps reveal that the journey of faith and formation unfolds gradually, often beginning in a place of striving—where we seek safety, belonging, purpose, or blessing in ways that are still shaped by fear or self-concern. As life stretches us through seasons of disruption, disillusionment, or honest questioning, we're invited into a deeper surrender—a letting go of the false attachments we've clung to for security, a surrender of the control that meant so much to us in our early years. It's in this sacred tension between striving and surrender that true transformation begins to take place because God stands in each threshold, holding us in the discomfort and darkness.

Slowly then, we can become more whole—less driven by fear or the need for approval, more anchored in a selfhood that is secure and surrendered, rooted in love, open to mystery, and attuned to the quiet presence of God.

The Path

Centuries ago, a woman wrote her story of spiritual transformation. In her day, women weren't encouraged to study, to write, or to engage spiritual matters in depth, but she did. Her name was Teresa Sánchez de Cepeda Dávila y Ahumada. She was born in 1515, a Spanish woman who'd eventually become known as St. Teresa of Ávila, the first female doctor of the church, as declared by Pope Paul VI in 1970. For me, there may be no more important voice than hers—a woman who faced abuse, persecution, and misogyny but whose courageous journey offers us a guide for our own. She recognized that there are some recognizable waypoints that we visit throughout our lives. And each offers us the possibility of further growth and maturation—and ultimately, our reorientation toward home once again.[11]

There are seven waypoints, or dwellings, as she calls them. I've named them using seven words that begin with *C*—curiosity, commitment, control, crisis, conversion, cruciformity, and communion. These anticipate the developmental stages of Erik Erickson and the stages of faith that James Fowler envisioned four centuries later, as well as the exceptional work of Janet Hagberg and Robert Guelich in their book, *The Critical Journey*.

St. Teresa's seven dwellings—along with Fowler's stages—trace a pattern of character integration and formation that mirrors Brueggemann's flow of orientation, disorientation, and reorientation, only in more detail. The journey begins with an early season of security, growth, and learning. This includes the stages I have labeled curiosity, commitment, and control. This first season provides a needed sense of safety, structure, and stability, although it can veer toward constriction and control. The journey continues with the middle season: doubt, disruption, and surrender. It's a long and winding path, with detours and backtracking, where we stumble and fall—where surrender is invited and deeper transformation takes place. This corresponds to the stages of crisis and conversion. Finally, we enter the final season, where a reoriented, God-shaped life emerges, rooted not in certainty but in love and union with God—cruciformity and communion.

Let's consider each critical threshold of the journey to maturity:

DWELLING (ST. TERESA)	FAITH STAGE (FOWLER)	DEVELOPMENTAL PSYCH THEME	CHARACTER TASK
1. Curiosity	Intuitive-Projective	Trust, imagination	Attachment and wonder
2. Commitment	Mythic-Literal	Moral structure, belonging	Early authenticity and good habits
3. Control	Synthetic-Conventional	Identity, performance	Competence with humility
4. Crisis	Transition to Reflective	Disruption, self-examination	Relinquishment and honest reckoning
5. Conversion	Individuative-Reflective	Self-authorship, integration	Inner integrity and mature authenticity
6. Cruciformity	Conjunctive	Relational depth, paradox	Compassionate, cruciform presence, and love
7. Communion	Universalizing	Union, legacy	Radiant love, being over doing

Stage 1: Curiosity

When we're newborns on the spiritual formation journey, we begin with a holy simplicity, characterized by childlike wonder and a sense of mystery. Whether we're young or old when we enter into faith, we embark on a quest to understand and reorient our world with Christ as our center. I recall how uncomplicated and magical faith seemed at first. If only I could have remained there!

As with our physical development, our early spiritual needs are basic: We need safety and trust; we need to be seen and known (what we described in chapter 1 as attachment, and what we discovered in chapter 4 as a core part of ancient, initiatory traditions). After all, the world gets complicated soon enough. But St. Teresa intuited a basic need beyond safety. Well before psychologists, she realized that God was *also* inviting us to experience delight, ease, wonder, and intimacy. She writes, "The soul . . . is none other than a garden in which the Beloved takes great delight."[12]

I sometimes think of this as a Garden of Eden phase, not meant to be rushed, inviting us to linger, to enjoy simple union and communion. And this is so very different from where some traditions begin, whether it's with an inordinate focus on what's most deeply wrong with you or with an urgent sense of what needs to be done. The first focuses on fixing you and the second on getting you to work.

Consider Jessica, who experienced both. She told me about "getting saved" through a campus ministry while she was still a freshman in college. She'd been told that she was a sinner in danger of hell but that God had provided a way to get right with him. Yet when she prayed to get right, she noted how she was immediately thrust into sharing Jesus with others. "I quickly learned that life for Jesus is the life of a worker bee," she said. "I needed to get right with Jesus, and then start getting others right with Jesus. Everything felt anxious and urgent—literally a matter of life and death." For Jessica's spiritual mentors, there was no time to linger in wonder or cultivate curiosity—only an urgent need for action and proclamation. As a result, Jessica explained that she spent the majority of her early days feeling like she was not doing enough or doing something wrong, and so she learned to hide her doubts, concerns, and failures.

Unfortunately, we see this too often today—to the detriment of our character formation. Busyness might produce compliance, but not Christlike character.

When we aren't invited to safely explore the lush garden of our hearts, as St. Teresa might say, or to experience the smile of God, our bodies and brains intuit that the world is unsafe—and they become vigilant. But building connection and cultivating curiosity are essential to growing lives of deep character. In fact, St. Teresa would say that, if we want to confront our sins and the world's pain truthfully, we need this early, cultivated sense of safety. Knowing that we're loved securely breeds honesty.

According to St. Teresa, there is no need to rush through this early season of the journey. We have all the time in the world to remain here, cultivating awe, wonder, and intimacy—enjoying the "deep, deep love of Jesus."[13] God isn't anxious or in a rush—nor should we be. Even still, just as a child must grow up and face the harsher realities of the world, so we cannot stay forever in this early season of wonder and simplicity.

Stage 2: Commitment

Think about a child in her earliest years beginning to explore her world. She takes her first steps toward a glowing fireplace, intrigued by the warmth and colors, only to be met by a kind and attuned mother who says, "Hot!" A good mother longs to cultivate her child's sense of wonder and confidence while providing the necessary boundaries.

And so it goes with spiritual development.

During this season of growing commitment, people's budding wonder and connection lead to a growing desire to move out into the world and live out their commitments. Just as a well-timed "no" and a hearty "yes!" (with attuned glances of concern and affirmation) help a child navigate the wild territory of their young hearts, so Jessica needed the guidance of an elder on her initiatory journey of faith. Though it didn't happen right away, she eventually found that in Jan—a woman in her midfifties who had navigated her own journey and would help guide Jessica as she moved through her early faith development.

It was in this season that Jessica finally started to slow down after her hurried start. She and Jan spent time together reading books, engaging questions, and asking, "What does it mean to follow Jesus?" Jessica felt seen and valued by Jan, and she grew in authentic faith. This is the safety, eldering, and anchoring in a sacred story we learned about in chapter 4, and it's so very necessary for spiritual development.

St. Teresa speaks of the importance of this early formation, with its need for attuned mentors, new insights, and a nascent intuition of what's good and what's not so good. "No matter how halfhearted such insights may be," she writes, "God rejoices whenever we learn what he is trying to teach us."[14] Early in childhood—and in our spiritual development—we're like sponges, taking in everything. But we need a good menu and a good mentor.

Character development suffers when our spiritual elders and mentors are too protective (attachment without authenticity), too permissive (authenticity without attachment), or too disengaged (no attachment or authenticity). But Jan was attuned, guiding Jessica to make wise decisions about what to engage and what to leave behind. A helper by nature, Jessica might have gotten overinvolved if it wasn't for Jan's wise counsel.

Stage 3: Control

Any parent of a teen knows that adolescence brings a slow shift in control as the child grows in independence. When their earliest needs have been met in childhood, this can be a beautiful movement: The young person goes beyond the safe boundaries of home into social relationships and school, where they continue to become themselves. If the story unfolds as it should, they remain confident even among pressures of social conformity, less likely to be tossed about in the winds of change or the storms of failure—not without pain or tears, of course—but with some resilience, because they are secure in their budding identity.

And yet as any parent of a teen knows, this isn't always how it plays out.

The same is true for our spiritual adolescence.

This is a crucial season, when growing confidence can lead to control and certainty—something we see in spades among abusive leaders, even Christian ones. Many of the most abusive spiritual leaders and systems I've seen appear to be stuck in this third-dwelling spirituality; they see control and certainty as a sort of spiritual destination, when in reality, infinitely more lies ahead. This is often, at the core, not intentional but unconscious, an act of survival amidst distressing dysregulation. But it comes with a cost.

Jessica wasn't immune to this.

Jessica's early introduction to faith was born in anxiety, and she couldn't shake the fear-based faith she was apprenticed into. Attracted by the seriousness and certainty of a popular local pastor, Jessica embraced a new tribe, a group with solid convictions and surefire takes on the crucial issues of the day. This mitigated her anxieties for a season—it even fostered unexpected confidence in her. Jessica took to social media to share her convictions with certainty, alienating some old friends. But at times, she'd become uncharacteristically combative and argumentative. In fact, when some of her new companions convinced her that Jan wasn't theologically sophisticated enough, Jessica ended their mentoring relationship.

Soon enough, Jessica married Rob, a man whose views she shared, and they had children and began to build a life together—but she couldn't shake a quiet restlessness within. She lamented being cut off from family and friends with different convictions. She missed Jan. She didn't always like how Rob treated her, especially when he used his theology to justify it. And her anxiety—it hadn't gone away but was secretly simmering within. These feelings shook her; she didn't understand why she had "plunged into disquiet,"[15] as St. Teresa put it, when she'd held her faith with such certainty for so long.

Stage 4: Crisis

Those who dare to journey forward learn that beyond control lies disorientation—a crisis that dismantles the old scaffolding of certainty. St. Teresa metaphorically likens this season to the collapse of a once-mighty Roman aqueduct that was masterfully constructed to be a conduit of much-needed water. Likewise, we craft coping mechanisms—even in the guise of theological and ecclesial systems—hoping they'll give us what we need. But they eventually crack and crumble too. God is often found in the wreckage.

What initiatory traditions, child psychologists, and faith development theorists agree on is this: Maturity requires that we learn to metabolize our suffering. Like we've talked about, this means staying with it, digesting it, processing it, even letting it mature us. But those stuck in the stage of "control" never learn to steward their pain. What happens, then, when life brings disappointment, disruption, doubt, disease, even a threat of death? What was Jessica to do with the persistent uneasiness inside her?

In desperation, Jessica called Jan one day, almost twelve years after their estrangement. Jan was now in her late sixties. Hearing Jan's familiar voice and joyful tears, Jessica felt her calcified heart begin to melt. Jessica named both the gifts of a season in which she'd found some belonging and certainty but also the loneliness and lack of fulfillment that accompanied it.

"No one sees me quite like you did, Jan," she said. "And I'm beginning to wonder what I believe anymore. The guy who led our community—well, he's been so harsh and controlling, and my husband has become the same way. I'm honestly scared at times."

Jan held space for Jessica's new questions, even helping her make some important decisions related to her relationships and boundaries. Jan knew that Jessica needed some hand-holding through this wilderness season—and a safe place to cry, at times, and perhaps even to scream.

Today, some call this stage a season of deconstruction. But whatever name it goes by, it invites character-deepening humility, and it requires an honest integration of our exiled ache—our painful emotions, our embodied sensations, our troubled thoughts, our besetting doubts, our spiritual malaise. A psalm of disorientation gives us an example of this reckoning:

> For my soul is full of troubles,
>   and my life draws near to Sheol.
> I am counted among those who go down to the Pit;
>   I am like those who have no help.
>
> PSALM 88:3-4, NRSVUE

It's scary—no one would disagree. And in this stage of crisis, there's often resistance—resistance to the losses that will come if we relinquish control, resistance to the uncertainty we'll feel if we dare to live our questions, resistance to voicing any doubts at all.

Yet, this time can be sacred too. Janet Hagberg and Robert Guelich describe this stage as the "Wall" in their book, *The Critical Journey*:

> The Wall, a dark and sacred place, reeks of God. In the Wall we are vulnerable enough to listen to what God says—whether it is in the guise of other people's voices, God's voice, or serendipitous experiences. Once we believe that God is in the midst of the darkness with us, it can be a transforming place. We don't necessarily get cured or erase our pain or become saints, but we learn how to embrace our pain, how to stay with it and learn what it is trying to teach us, how to look fear in the face and keep moving into it.[16]

The Wall meets us in different ways: doubt, despair, disease, diagnoses, disillusionment, disorientation, distress, deconstruction, dullness of faith. Whatever form it takes, it invites deep wrestling. Here, like the Israelites, we must leave the clarity Sinai offered and enter into the uncertain depths of the wilderness. It's not faithlessness, but faithful wrestling.

Jessica was at a wall. And she was scared. She was questioning everything now—the early scare tactics of her first mentors, the unapologetic certainty of her previous tribe, the high control exerted by Rob in her marriage. She wondered what was true. Everything felt like it was falling apart.

Stage 5: Conversion

Jessica began to understand why she was so drawn to certainty and a sense of belonging. In her desire to mitigate her anxiety and fill her core needs, she had sought security in rock-solid convictions and in a high-control environment. But she was ultimately disappointed when they led not to union with God, but to self-righteousness and growing dissatisfaction. Was it all worthless? Had she been duped? Thankfully, in Jan's presence, she felt safe and held. And it seemed that Jan knew and embodied a larger story that could hold even Jessica's unraveling.

In this season of maturation, what feels like crisis reveals itself as profoundly transformational. St. Teresa likens it to the caterpillar and the chrysalis—a place of hidden metamorphosis and deeper conversion. In early spiritual life, we're similar to the caterpillar, who crawls along the ground, consuming everything in sight. That's all we know. But because we're God's image bearers, we long for so much more. We're not made to crawl; we're made to fly.

But first, a radical interior conversion needs to take place.

For the caterpillar, this happens in the chrysalis stage of metamorphosis, when it undergoes complete cellular transformation. Its old structure is broken down into a kind of biological soup. From this dissolution, imaginal cells activate and guide the formation of a radically new creature—the butterfly. When its transformation is complete, the butterfly pushes through the chrysalis, unfolds its delicate wings, and—drawing strength from the sun—takes flight into a life it could never have imagined from the ground.

Jan provided a safe, chrysalis space for Jessica to begin to wrestle with God amidst her many losses and questions. Jessica made courageous decisions during this time, for the sake of her own selfhood, her marriage, even her faltering faith. Because she was held tenderly in this space, Jessica found the struggle becoming less scary—and even strangely freeing. Knowing she was held securely allowed her to let go of what wouldn't serve growth and transformation in this season; instead, she could embrace new relationships, new ways of understanding, and new practices. She did hard things she had never imagined doing, surprising herself with her courage and resilience.

The butterfly is a reminder to us that true transformation requires both death and re-formation. This conversion process is similar to the ripening we talked about in earlier chapters. Many people attempt performative ripening—maturing without real change and transformation. Yet those who ultimately surrender to a grace-filled transformation discover an emerging authenticity and inner integration, a wholeness that renders the old caterpillar life small by comparison.

Stage 6: Cruciformity

Jessica's initiatory journey through her own chrysalis of surrender and transformation wasn't quick or painless. It required the dismantling of many beliefs she'd once counted as sturdy and true, including the perception of her marriage. With the attuned support of Jan and others in her community, Jessica wrestled with her questions for more than a decade, bringing her faith and her marriage to the brink. But it was Jessica's faithfulness to this mysterious and disorienting process—even her faith that God was at the very center of it—that eventually awakened her husband, Rob, too. Later, they would acknowledge that, while from the outside their marriage had looked strong, it needed to be dismantled and rebuilt on a foundation of mutual respect and trust. Only then could it flourish and endure.

This is the long, cruciform journey toward authentic maturity.

The cruciform shape of a life is patterned after the dying and rising of Jesus. This is the sacred story. And anyone who has navigated disorientation and come out the other side knows something of its redemptive shape. According to Paul, the fruits of "love, joy, peace, patience, kindness, goodness, faithfulness, gentleness, and self-control" grow in those who "live by the Spirit" (Galatians 5:22-23, 25). It's a slow walk, to be sure. And it's a winding wilderness journey.

In her writings, St. Teresa does not promise escape from suffering; instead, she bears witness to a deeper anchoring in God amidst the uproar of life. She reveals how safety, eldering, community, and a sacred story ground those who dare to walk the cruciform way of Jesus. This is not a mystical ascent but an embodied faith, forged in the fire of everyday trials and interior wrestling. And yet through it all, there is a steady, growing union with Christ.

Stage 7: Communion

Throughout the Christian tradition, there is universal agreement that a life in the Spirit will culminate in union and communion with God—a foretaste, even now, of what we'll experience fully when Jesus returns to make all things new (Revelation 21:5).

This is a radical evolution of the self beyond earlier patterns of striving, certainty, and control. What once manifested as performative faith—striving to prove, promote, or perfect oneself—now gives way to effortless presence, a life of spaciousness marked by communion rather than control.

Such a person doesn't go looking for suffering but is unafraid of it. Like Jesus on the cross, this person looks not to hold grudges but to forgive lavishly.

Through the years, Jan remained a steady source of wisdom and guidance for Jessica. And one day, decades after they first met, Jessica spoke at Jan's funeral. Her tears flowed uninterrupted, a testimony to Jan's faithful presence in her life. In her last years, Jan seemed to live with an otherworldly peace while, at the same time, remaining remarkably grounded and involved in the affairs of life. Jan was known as *Immah* to Jessica's kids, a play on a Hebrew term of affection for a close maternal figure.

Now Jessica had become the elder to other women. She was a woman who held space—without force or demand—stewarding suffering and creating the kind of safety so vital to the maturation of others. She now held the map, in her body, of a lived story of orientation, disorientation, and reorientation. She'd traversed St. Teresa's path herself.

Theologian Cornelius Plantinga describes a flourishing, spiritually whole person this way:

> She longs for God and the beauty of God, for Christ and Christlikeness, for the dynamite of the Holy Spirit and spiritual maturity. . . . She longs for other human beings: she wants to love them and to be loved by them. She hungers for social justice. She longs for nature, for its beauties and graces. . . . She is a person of character consistency, a person who rings true wherever you tap her. She keeps promises. She

> weeps with those who weep and, perhaps more impressively, rejoices with those who rejoice. She does all these things in ways that express her own personality and culture but also a general "mind of Christ" that is cross-culturally unmistakable.[17]

Jan and Jessica went on this journey—a journey that required them to navigate challenging passages but that matured them into wholeness.

St. Teresa did as well.

And I, for one, am grateful for those who've taken it—leaving trail markers behind. I, too, long for the kind of life that flourishes. I long to become myself, as they did.

Who We Are . . . in God

There is no way to grow other than by going out into the world, where we'll learn the necessary lessons for a reoriented life. It's how true character is formed. The poet Mary Oliver names this reality in her book *Upstream*, writing, "In the beginning I was so young and such a stranger to myself I hardly existed. I had to go out into the world and see it and hear it and react to it, before I knew at all who I was, what I was, what I wanted to be."[18]

The long journey home to ourselves and to God is never linear.

It meanders through seasons of clarity and collapse, belonging and bewilderment, scaling thrilling heights and plumbing new depths. But when we glimpse the pattern—from curiosity to communion, from suffering to surrender—we begin to trust that even the wilderness seasons are not wasted. They are, in fact, necessary initiations in a journey God will bring to completion through Jesus (Philippians 1:6).

The destination, as St. Teresa reminds us, is not some distant spiritual trophy, but the deep recognition that we are already home in God. The soul becomes quiet. Love becomes the center. And life, once governed by effort and performance, flows more freely from presence, union, and joy.

This is what the ancients meant by character transformation—not becoming someone else but finally becoming who we are in God.

And so, dear friends,

May you trust the long road of becoming—
with its twists and thresholds, its wonder and weariness,
knowing that growth unfolds not in haste,
but through seasons of orientation, disorientation, and slow reorientation.

May you be patient with the parts of you still in process—
the controlling you, the fearful you, the faltering you,
and may you meet them not with shame, but with compassion and grace.

May you learn to walk with ancient maps in hand—
guided by saints, prophets, and poets—and elders among us,
who knew that the path to union is not upward, but downward,
through suffering, surrender, and the slow ripening of love.

May you find courage to let go of what no longer serves you,
and space to receive what is deeper, quieter, and more true—
a life no longer centered in piety or performance,
but grounded in God, rooted in love, and open to mystery.

And may you come to know—
not just believe, but deeply know—
that the home you've been seeking is not far off,
but within you, all along,
where Christ dwells and calls you to be.

RESOURCES

- St. Teresa of Ávila, trans. Mirabai Starr, *The Interior Castle*
- Walter Brueggemann, *The Psalms and the Life of Faith*
- James W. Fowler, *Stages of Faith: The Psychology of Human Development and the Quest for Meaning*
- Janet O. Hagberg and Robert A. Guelich, *The Critical Journey: Stages in the Life of Faith*

REFLECTION

1. When you look back over your life of faith, where do you see seasons of orientation (clarity, belonging, confidence), disorientation (loss, doubt, disruption), and reorientation (new depth, surrendered trust)? Where do you see yourself right now?
2. Which of St. Teresa's stages or "C words" (curiosity, commitment, control, crisis, conversion, cruciformity, communion) best names your current season? What in your life makes you say that?
3. Where are you clinging to control, certainty, or performance in ways that may have served you in an earlier stage but now feel constricting or exhausting?
4. What forms of suffering, disappointment, or confusion are you currently facing? What might change if you saw these not as proof

of failure, but as invitations into deeper maturation and union with God?

5. Who are the "elders" (living or dead, whether mentors, writers, or saints) whose stories give you courage in your current stage? What might it look like to follow their guidance more closely right now?

PRACTICE

Cultivating Reorientation for the Sake of Character Change

This exercise can be done in twenty to thirty minutes with a journal. It's meant to help you locate yourself, name what you need, and discern how your maturation might unfold.

STEP 1: GROUND YOURSELF

Find a comfortable place, breathing slowly and gently for a minute or two.

Reflect on the following passage:

> You have searched me, LORD,
> and you know me.
> You know when I sit and when I rise;
> you perceive my thoughts from afar.
> You discern my going out and my lying down;
> you are familiar with all my ways.
>
> PSALM 139:1-3

STEP 2: LOOK BACK—TRACE THE ROAD SO FAR

Draw a simple line across a page to represent your spiritual/life journey. Make five to seven hash marks to represent key moments or seasons, and write a brief summation next to each mark (e.g., "college conversion," "life-changing retreat," "rupture in close friendship," "marriage issues begin," "youngest child's rebellion," "new life-giving reading group," etc.).

Then, next to each one, write the letter (O, D, or R) that best fits that season:

O—Orientation (clarity, stability, belonging)

D—Disorientation (loss, confusion, disruption)

R—Reorientation (new depth, growing meaning, surprising joy)

Consider:

- Is there a particular moment, movement, or pattern that stands out?
- Over the course of your life, in which season have you spent the most time?

STEP 3: LOCATE YOUR PRESENT STAGE

Now look at St. Teresa's seven waypoints. Choose the one that best fits this current season:

Curiosity—early wonder, questions, attraction

Commitment—strong belonging, clear boundaries, zeal

Control—certainty, performance, identity built on being right or effective

Crisis—the Wall, disillusionment, doubt, dryness, disruption

Conversion—hidden re-forming, surrender, imaginal "chrysalis" work

Cruciformity—deeper union, shared suffering, growing compassion

Communion—quiet, spacious, non-anxious love and presence

Write a few lines reflecting on your life right now:

This season feels like ____ because ________________________. When I read the list above, the features that feel familiar in this season are ________________________________

____.

STEP 4: ASK THREE QUESTIONS FOR THIS SEASON

Under that description, answer these questions:

1. What is this stage inviting you to *let go of* (beliefs, behaviors, identities, relationships to control)?
2. What is this stage inviting you to *receive* (support, practices, truths, companions)?
3. What kind of maturation might be happening beneath the surface (deeper trust, humility, compassion, differentiation, courage, openness to mystery)—even if you can't see transformation yet?

If it helps, imagine an elder like St. Teresa, James Fowler, Walter Brueggemann, Jan, or a trusted mentor gently naming what this season is "for" in your life. What would they observe or say?

STEP 5: NAME WHAT YOU NEED NOW

Finish by writing two simple, concrete next steps:

- One practice that fits this stage

  Curiosity: wonder, imaginative prayer, childlike gratitude

  Commitment: basic rhythms, learning in community, finding belonging

  Control: identifying egoistic tendencies, identifying gifts, pursuing goals

  Crisis: lament, therapy/spiritual direction, acknowledging wounds/disappointment

  Conversion: silence, Sabbath, saying no to old roles, slower pace

  Cruciformity: compassionate service, presence with suffering, forgiving work

  Communion: hiddenness, mentoring others, radical gentleness

- One relational move

    reaching out to a mentor or spiritual director

    sharing honestly with a trusted friend

    joining (or leaving) a specific community or role

    asking someone (attuned therapist, spiritual director, pastoral counselor) to walk with you as you face your "Wall"

Write down these intentions as a short prayer:

In this season of ______________________, I sense you inviting me to let go of ______________________ and receive ______________________. Give me courage to take this next step: __________________________________ ____.

Close by slowly meditating on Philippians 1:6: "You who began a good work in me will carry it on to completion . . ."

Let that be the benediction wherever you are on the map—unfinished, yes, but deeply held.

PART 3

the transformation of character

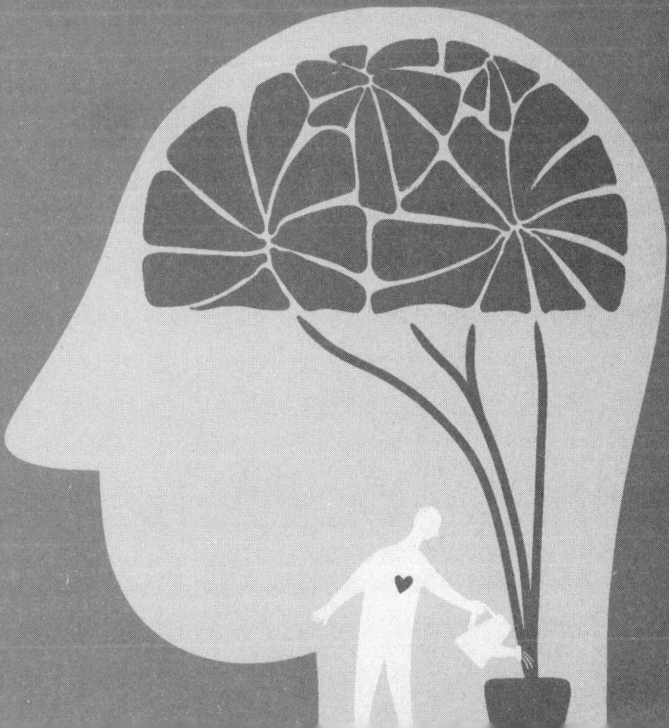

Faith, hope, and love
form the gravitational center of the Christian life—
not vague aspirations,
but the very telos of character,
the soul's true orientation.
Faith
anchors us in trust,
loosening our grip on control,
freeing us to live not by striving,
but by surrender—
not from fear,
but from the quiet, grounded strength of being held.
Hope
roots us in a future not yet seen,
resisting the gravity of cynicism,
of despair.
It lifts our eyes,
teaches us to breathe
when the way is hidden
and the heart is tired.

Love—

the greatest of these—
is the radiant overflow
of a life no longer turned inward in fear,
but opened wide
to communion,
connection,
compassion.
Together,
they are not merely virtues,
but the shape of a soul made whole—
the fruit of a life
formed in Christ,
fully human,
fully alive.

CHAPTER 7

renewed

Grounding Faith in an Age of Fight, Fear, and Fix

Help me to journey beyond the familiar and into the unknown.
Give me the faith to leave old ways and break fresh ground with you.
Christ of the mysteries,
I trust you to be stronger than each storm within me.
I will trust in the darkness and know
that my times, even now, are in your hand.
ATTRIBUTED TO ST. BRENDAN THE NAVIGATOR, SIXTH CENTURY

Be transformed by the renewing of your mind.
ROMANS 12:2

Maddie grew up in a home where responsibility quietly eclipsed relationship. Her parents were competent, driven professionals who valued order, discipline, and achievement, but they lacked the time—or perhaps the emotional capacity—to tend to her inner world. Maddie learned early that being good, capable, and self-sufficient was the safest way to belong. Her feelings learned to wait.

Luis's home was shaped by a very different kind of absence. His childhood was marked by chaos and volatility, punctuated by vicious fights between his mother and stepfather. He learned to stay alert, quietly carrying his sadness and anger while trying to anticipate the next emotional storm. Where Maddie learned restraint, Luis learned reactivity.

Maddie excelled in college and graduate school. She was sharp and steady, but she also noticed a growing scrupulosity. Her head became her enemy. Therapy became the first place where her inner life was welcomed, and what followed was a season of long-suppressed emotion finally given voice.

Luis, meanwhile, skipped college and joined his uncle in a local moving business. His emotions surged and crashed until he met Alvin, who offered him something he had never known: a way to manage the inner chaos through clarity and cognitive mastery. Luis spent the next decade immersed in courses offered through a Bible institute, finding steadiness in ideas while relegating his conflicted emotions to the basement of his psyche.

Each eventually found a Christian community that affirmed their way of being in the world. Maddie's expressiveness was named authenticity. Luis's theological certainty was named faithfulness. And in real ways, both changed. But this would not be the end of their spiritual journeys.

Both Maddie and Luis eventually hit a wall. Amidst their disorientation, they came to see that, though they had learned to cope by relying on their head or heart, just getting by was a cheap substitute for real, wholehearted transformation. And they realized that faithful change would not require them to sacrifice either one—they needed both for the lasting renewal they longed for.

I've seen versions of Maddie's and Luis's stories over and again throughout the years, even in my own. When it comes to living from our head or our heart, we're prone to swing from one extreme to another. The emotional family drama of my earliest years led me into a spiritual community that prized order and rationality. But after spending years there, I was still experiencing stagnation from emotional disconnection. This led me to seek a more therapeutic community, and this swing led to unvarnished emotionalism. Looking back, I remember the sense of certainty I felt in each space, believing I'd discovered the right way to be faithful and true. I see that same certainty in communities—spiritual and otherwise—that prize one aspect of a person over the whole.

Maddie and Luis appear to have taken opposite paths, yet their stories share a common thread. In different ways, both were pulled toward a particular way of being human. Maddie's community believed that the heart was the key: human flourishing emerged through emotional connectedness and relational transparency. Luis's assumed that the head was most important: flourishing followed careful study, doctrinal integrity, and right living. Both had Scripture to back them up. And both felt quite confident that they were faithfully growing into more mature Christians.

Is faithfulness a matter of the head or the heart?

What Hemisphere Are You Living In?

The unfortunate division between head and heart, witnessed throughout the history of the church, makes sense when you consider the brain. Maybe you've heard that it has two hemispheres—the left and the right. You may not realize, however, that they represent not just different functions but different ways of attending to the world. The left brain seeks certainty and coherence, while the right brain longs for connection and lived experience.

How does one of the two become dominant to the exclusion of the other?

Hemispheric dominance is often less about temperament and more about formation. The stories we inherit and the communities that shape us tend to reward certain ways of attending to the world while discouraging others. In some settings, emotional restraint, certainty, and cognitive mastery are praised as virtues. Though Luis's early formation was shaped in chaos, he gravitated toward a more rational, left-brained faith because it seemed to settle him (at least for a while). For him, being transformed by the renewing of his mind meant mastering his feelings with cognitive certainty—something that worked for a season, as he shifted from chaos to control.

In other settings, expressiveness, emotional intensity, and immediacy are seen as signs of emotional and spiritual health. Over time, these repeated reinforcements train the mind to rely disproportionately on the right hemisphere. Maddie experienced an expansion of her world as she shifted from left-brained dominance into the more spacious and relational realm of the right. The renewal she experienced was a reconnection to her heart.

It's not just individuals who emphasize one way of showing up in the world. You've seen these divisions become mottos of churches, organizations, perhaps even people you know.

- "Right belief leads to right living."
- "Authentic relationships are what matter most."
- "Truth over feelings—always."
- "If we're not changing the world, we're missing the point."
- "Healing happens when you finally let it all out."

We build whole churches and movements out of these slogans, with all sorts of implications for character formation to boot. Blind to the limits of our own way of seeing, we elevate a God-given part of us in lieu of the whole.

Even more, we are tempted to believe we've landed on the one and only right path.

Both brain hemispheres are crucial, designed to work as partners, each offering a different way of attending to reality. As Iain McGilchrist reminds us, the right hemisphere is meant to take a lead role, opening us to the world as living, relational, and whole; the left contributes by analyzing, categorizing, and bringing clarity to what the right perceives.[1] However, when we rely too much on one viewpoint—especially under stress—we can begin to live from a place of one-sided dominance rather than whole-brained integration.

As both Maddie and Luis realized over time, each hemisphere of the brain is vulnerable to distortion when asked to do more than it was meant to. The left hemisphere excels at clarity, categorization, and problem-solving. But when it becomes the dominant pattern—especially in response to threat or chaos—it can harden into control, mistaking certainty for wisdom and explanation for transformation. The left hemisphere becomes problematic, not because it is analytical, but because it forgets that it exists in relationship, designed to serve a larger way of knowing.

The right hemisphere, for its part, is oriented toward presence, context, and embodied relationship. It helps us sense meaning rather than define it, remain open to mystery, and stay attuned to what is unfolding in the moment. Yet when the right hemisphere becomes disconnected from the left, we might experience intensity without integration, or emotional immersion without a sense of orientation or larger perspective-taking. Neither the right nor the left was ever meant to carry the whole on its own.

Renewal, as Scripture imagines it, is not found in choosing one side over the other. It is not a battle between head and heart but the construction of a harmonious relationship between two necessary ways of knowing. The integration and transformation we long for do not come from choosing one side over the other, but from seeking to develop a new mind—a whole way of seeing that invites every part of us to the table.

Transformation of the Mind

When we talk about the brain, we mean the physical organ—an astonishing three-pound neural network inside our skull. But when Scripture speaks of the "mind," it means something larger. The mind is not just tissue and circuitry; it is the way we see the world. The brain makes thinking possible. But the mind reflects how we are attending. And what we attend to, again and again, slowly shapes who we become.[2]

This helps us get to what the apostle Paul meant when he called the Roman church to be "transformed by the renewing of your mind" (Romans 12:2). It's one of Paul's great clues to transformation, but what's fascinating is that he doesn't spend the chapter telling his Roman audience what they should *know*. There is no division of head and heart here. There is no split between ideas and action. For Paul, the "mind" is not a detached faculty, but the lens through which the whole person lives and acts. This transformation is about the renewal of your center of gravity, in one sense—or put another way, a renewal of your way of seeing. In a divided world and with a sometimes-divided brain, it's about a renewed sense of wholeness.

The apostle Paul writes about the renewal of the mind in Romans 12 during a time when people were seeing in a particular way—through a lens of superiority. This was the dilemma: The Roman church was made up of Gentile and Jewish Christians who were at odds with one another and their surrounding culture. These ethnic divisions led to a desire for status and cultural power, as well as presumption and condescension between believers. But Paul offers a new vision, empowered by a new mind. In fact, he clarifies what he means by the renewing of the mind just one verse later: "Think of yourself with sober judgment, in accordance with the faith God has distributed to each of you" (verse 3). He is not proposing an enlightened new theology but a life of sobriety and humility, manifesting in self-giving love.

Maybe you're beginning to see, too, that this renewal of the mind is not so much about superiority—right doctrine, right worship, right feelings, right mission, right relationships—but a *whole* new way of seeing, a new way of being, what Paul elsewhere calls "the mind of Christ" (1 Corinthians 2:16).

A New Mind

You know the feeling—you might be sitting at your desk with your laptop open and yet forget why you opened it in the first place. You might open your fridge only to blank on what you needed. When they were young, my daughters used to call it brain freeze. While most people experience these brief mental lapses from time to time, when the human psyche is under chronic stress, it tends to compartmentalize and dis-integrate in even more significant ways. This disconnection shows up, not only in the sense of division between the two hemispheres of our mind but in all sorts of internal fragmentation, particularly when we're overwhelmed or threatened.

I sometimes describe a frazzled inner world as an orchestra

without a conductor. Parts of you feel like they're in conflict. There is a version of you that shows up to church, and another that secretly looks at pornography. There's a part of you that beats yourself up, and another that feels like you've got it all figured out. There's a part of you that holds your baby tenderly, and another that quietly wonders whether you were ever meant to become a mother. If you're reading this and nodding in recognition, you're not broken—you're human.

But like an orchestra without a conductor, that fragmentation can become chaotic. Tubas compete with trumpets, trombones drown out flutes, cymbals crash at inopportune moments—each instrument playing at its own tempo and volume, none listening for the whole.

What's needed in such moments is not the silencing of instruments, but coordination—something that can hold the whole, notice what's happening, and gently bring things back into relationship. This is where the capacities we associate with the mind come into play, which are supported in the brain by the prefrontal cortex (PFC).

As we saw in chapter 3, the PFC is deeply involved in attention, reflection, impulse regulation, and perspective taking. Rather than being the conductor, it helps make conducting possible. It supports the mind's capacity to pause, to observe competing impulses without immediately obeying them, and to choose how we respond. When these capabilities are accessible—when we are regulated enough—we are able to inhabit a more spacious inner posture, one marked by curiosity, compassion, and discernment.

In this sense, the PFC does not rule the orchestra; it helps us hear it. It creates the conditions under which leadership can emerge—not the dominance of one part over the others, but a grounded, integrated presence that can let them all be heard in harmony. Through this renewed posture of mind, we learn to pay attention and engage intentionally, fostering pathways of humility, generosity, love, mutuality, and wholeness—repatterning not only the brain but also our lives. Over time, the renewed mind supports a growing capacity to live from our true self, rather than letting anxious, reactive, or controlling parts seize the wheel.

We need the capacities supported by the PFC accessible and attuned—especially when certain instruments in our inner orchestra begin to dominate or when parts of us are in conflict. When we are able to slow down and attend in this way, we gain something crucial: the ability to observe rather than immediately react, to remain present without being overtaken by a particular impulse. The writer of Proverbs offers this wise counsel: "Better a patient person than a warrior, one with self-control than one who takes a city" (Proverbs 16:32). And Paul calls self-control a fruit of the Spirit (Galatians 5:22-23).

This is not a cold or detached form of control, but a spacious kind of seeing that allows us to notice what is happening internally without being flooded by it. For this reason, the prefrontal cortex is closely associated with curiosity, compassion, perspective, and choice—capacities that many Christian traditions recognize as expressions of the "true self."

When I was stuck in a left-brain dominant season of intellectual certainty and rational superiority, I had no sense of what was happening within, nor a sense of my impact on others. Early on in my counseling journey, a kind classmate took me aside and said, "Chuck, this may be hard to hear, but until now I've experienced you as arrogant, distant, and condescending." It was disheartening at first, but my initial defensiveness relaxed into curiosity. The community was safe enough to hold me in that season. As my PFC became more resourceful, I sensed what my fellow student said was true—for too long I'd lived ungrounded, in fight-or-flight, my actions reflecting my body's chronic state of stress.

However, instead of blessing my left-brained capacities as a gift when they were regulated, I dismissed them. I divided head and heart—and chose heart. A few years later someone else came to me and shared something that stunned me: "Chuck, I hesitate to say this because you care so deeply, but I sense that you and your community only include folks who you consider emotionally in touch. It's like you're the enlightened ones, and the rest of us just don't get it. It hurts me." This honest feedback led me, once and for all, to step into a new way of seeing, which blessed both my left- and right-brained gifts and capacities, inviting them into a harmonious wholeness. This changed how I engaged with others too. My hope today is that I am more *mind*-ful than I used to be.

Maybe you, too, can begin to notice the moments when your inner orchestra narrows—when one instrument takes over and drowns out the rest. You might sense it in your body as a tightening in your chest, or a subtle urgency to fix, explain, withdraw, or prove yourself. Can you slow down long enough to notice the shift?

When we pause in this way, even briefly, we sense a widening within. The small turn from judgment to curiosity creates just enough space for the mind to do what it does best when it is resourced: to hold complexity, to listen across difference, and to respond rather than react. Slowly, often beneath our awareness, the orchestra begins to find its rhythm again. No instrument is exiled or forced into silence. And from that growing coherence emerges a quieter, steadier way of being—one less driven by fear or control, and more shaped by presence, humility, and love.

Grounded Faith

I long for this grounded faith, anchored amidst internal and external storms. Rather than being pulled in different directions and feeling inner fragmentation, I want to experience wholeness and peace. I long for this surrendered trust, not prone to self-sufficiency but resting in God's Spirit leading from within.

But I suspect that you and I are susceptible to the same kinds of problems the apostle Paul saw. We tend to "conform to the pattern of the world" rather than being transformed by the renewing of our minds (Romans 12:2). We are prone to patterns of superiority and certainty. We tend to elevate head or heart, maybe even requiring others to choose too. We're inclined, as we've seen in previous chapters, to live in reflexive responses like fight-or-flight. Ultimately, we're "conformed" to frazzled rather than faithful patterns.

Paul was writing in the first century, so he didn't have the language of nervous systems to inform him. But he did have a remarkably embodied understanding of human transformation. When he urges believers to "present your bodies as a living sacrifice" (Romans 12:1, ESV), he is not calling for heroic self-denial or spiritualized self-harm. He is inviting a reorientation of the whole person—body included—away from patterns of self-protection and self-sufficiency, toward a posture of faith and trust. In nervous-system terms, Paul is describing a movement away from chronic vigilance, rivalry, and striving, toward a settled offering of oneself from a place of safety and security.

This is what makes the rest of Romans 12 sing. Because what comes after his call to renew our minds is not a detached treatise but a vision of whole-person character transformation, with strong echoes of Paul's Christ hymn (Philippians 2:6-11) and the beatitudes

(Matthew 5:3-12)—words to shape a new imagination, a new way of being in the world. This was no mere faith of mental assent or emotional awakening; this was deep trust, yielding embodied living, women and men animated by the mind of Christ.

This is a surrendered life, a life of grounded and secure faith, no longer looking to dominate, elevate, subjugate, or eliminate. This is a wholehearted life, no longer looking to divide but to include.

How do you know you're making the shift from chaos to conductor? How do you know when you're no longer being carried by one dominant way of attending to the world and living from a more grounded center?

Internally, this move to a wider perspective may feel like a deeper awareness of parts in conflict, accompanied by a slow, growing curiosity about reflexive reactions, instinctual defenses, and long-standing patterns of hierarchy within us. Rather than rushing to resolve these tensions, we begin by noticing them.

Relationally, this posture shows up in simple but consequential ways. In conversation, we learn to pause and attend to what is happening within us before responding. Engaging these integrative capacities, we may find ourselves able to say, "I can see now how I became reactive. An old part of me that needs to be right took over, and I defaulted to fight rather than curiosity. I'm sorry." Such moments mark not perfection, but the quiet work of renewal.

Rarely does this shift announce itself with certainty or confidence. In fact, one of its clearest signs is a softening rather than a strengthening of conviction. The need to prove, persuade, or perform begins to loosen. Defenses dissolve. Resistances relax. What emerges instead is a quiet capacity to stay—with yourself, with others, and with complexity—without rushing to resolution. It's not that you abandon conviction, but you relax certainty. The late British missionary-theologian Lesslie Newbigin called it "proper confidence."[3]

This grounded place is not emotionally flat, nor is it intellectually rigid. You still think clearly. You still feel deeply. But neither thinking nor feeling is driving the whole. Because you're grounded in your true self, you have access to parts of you that sense, feel, discern, clarify, fear, anticipate, and more—but these parts no longer need to take over, because you (guided by the Spirit within you) are conducting the orchestra. You can speak on behalf of these parts of yourself without becoming conflated with them.

You begin to notice a widening inside—more space between impulse and action, more patience with ambiguity, more humility about what you know and do not know. The question subtly changes from "Am I right?" to "Am I present?"

Wholehearted Faith

Divided people tend to create divided worlds. But whole people—those learning to live from a grounded and integrated center—foster the kind of wholeness Paul imagines in Romans 12. His vision is not of uniformity or competition, but of a body made up of many members, each distinct, each necessary, each belonging to the others:

> Just as each of us has one body with many members, and these members do not all have the same function, so in Christ we, though many, form one body, and each member belongs to all the others. We have different gifts, according to the grace given to each of us.
>
> ROMANS 12:4-6

This is not merely a metaphor for church structure; it is a vision of mature humanity. A community shaped by renewed minds does not organize itself around comparison, superiority, or the need to be right. It is not driven by the anxious question, *Who has the purest faith?* but by a far more searching one: *What kind of people are we becoming? And what kind of life is being generated in and through us?*

In a season marked by scandal, abuse, and the exposure of long-hidden fractures within the church, this question matters deeply. Too often, faith has been measured by certainty of belief, emotional intensity, or visible impact—while the quieter fruits of humility, mercy, self-control, gentleness, and joy have been neglected or dismissed. A grounded faith calls us back to a different metric. Not how forcefully we defend our position, but how faithfully we embody love. Not how impressive our language is, but how trustworthy our lives are.

This renewal, in the end, is not merely about retuning a nervous system but reshaping the roots of our character. Like a tree drawing water from deeper soil, a renewed mind sinks beneath reactive patterns and anxious striving into a steadier source of life. As those roots deepen, the trunk strengthens—less brittle, less easily bent by cultural winds of outrage or certainty. And over time, fruit appears: not manufactured performance, but the kind of embodied love Paul describes—sincere, patient, hospitable, and devoted to the good of others (Romans 12:9-13). What is visible above ground is sustained by a hidden integration within, which you're learning to cultivate. And that's good news for you, for all of us, because your good fruit will abundantly bless you and those around you.

And so, once again, dear friends,

May you come to know a faith
that does not require you to choose
between thinking and feeling,
certainty and openness,
clarity and compassion.

May you be released from the exhausting task
of proving that your way of seeing
is the right one,
the enlightened one,
the faithful one.

May your mind be renewed
not by sharper arguments
or louder emotions,
but by a growing capacity
to remain present
to what is happening within you
and between you and others.

May your body learn again
that it is safe to rest—
safe to breathe more deeply,
safe to soften its vigilance,
safe to loosen its grip on certainty and defense.

May the Spirit of God meet you
in that quiet, centered place

where your thoughts no longer have to dominate,
your emotions no longer have to overwhelm,
and every part of you is welcome
without being in charge.

May you grow into the mind of Christ:
a mind shaped by humility rather than superiority,
by generosity rather than fear,
by love that is strong enough
to hold complexity without fracture.

And when you lose your ground—as you will—
may you return again and again
to the One who holds you,
who conducts the whole of your life with mercy,
and who is patiently renewing you
from the inside out.
Amen.

RESOURCES

- David G. Benner, *Surrender to Love: Discovering the Heart of Christian Spirituality*
- Iain McGilchrist, *Ways of Attending: How Our Divided Brain Constructs the World*
- Nicholas Rowe and Sheila Wise Rowe, *Healing Leadership Trauma: Finding Emotional Health and Helping Others Flourish*
- Matt Tebbe and Ben Sternke, *Having the Mind of Christ: Eight Axioms to Cultivate a Robust Faith*

REFLECTION

1. As you consider Maddie's, Luis's, and Chuck's stories, what aspects resonate with you?
2. How would you describe yourself through the lens of left-brain dominance or right brain dominance? What features of either show up in your life? What are the positives? The challenges?
3. If you were to honestly assess what you've been "conformed to," what would you name? What parts of you have become overly dominant? How has this emphasis kept you from seeing the perspective of another part of you or even another person?
4. How have you experienced greater connection to your "true self" within? How has this allowed you to gain a wider perspective? When you consider your "inner orchestra," what parts of yourself do you notice demanding the most attention? How can you show them attention and kindness without becoming stuck there?
5. Consider an organization, church, or institution that you know—and consider its fruit through the lens of Romans 12. How does it reflect the characteristics Paul describes? How might it be missing the mark? What does it tend to prioritize?

PRACTICE

Cultivating a Renewed Mind for the Sake of Character Change

Learning to Notice, Hold, and Re-center

This is a practice of noticing—of becoming curious about *how* you are attending to the world, especially when you feel pulled toward certainty, intensity, withdrawal, control, or something else. Think of it as a way of gently re-centering your inner life so that no single part of you has to carry the whole. By shifting your way of seeing, you slowly reshape your character.

You might return to this practice when you feel reactive, overly certain, emotionally flooded, or disconnected—or simply when you want to grow in a more grounded and embodied faith.

STEP 1: BEGIN WHERE YOU ARE

Find a comfortable posture and take a few slow breaths. You don't need to change anything—just notice.

Ask yourself quietly:

- *What feels most present in me right now?*

Not what *should* be present. Not what you think God wants. Simply what is.

You might notice thoughts racing, emotions rising, a tight jaw, a heavy chest, or a sense of urgency to do something. Let whatever you notice be there without judgment.

This is already the beginning of renewal: attention without correction.

STEP 2: NOTICE YOUR PULL

Now gently ask yourself:

- *When I'm not grounded and centered, what urges or pulls within tend to come forward?*

You're not choosing between right and wrong here—only noticing tendencies.

Simply name what you notice:

I notice a part of me that tends to dominate conversation.

I sense that I need to be dramatic to get my point across.

I see that I disappear in order to avoid conflict.

This isn't about what you're doing wrong. Each tendency emerged to help you survive and belong.

STEP 3: MAKE SPACE FOR THE WHOLE

Now imagine yourself stepping back just a little—you are not moving away from these parts, just observing them from a place of care and perspective.

You might say:

I notice these parts of me, and I am more than any one of them.

This is not disconnection; it's containment.

You're allowing your mind—the part of you capable of reflection, curiosity, and perspective—to behold the whole inner scene.

If it helps, place a hand on your chest or belly as a reminder that this awareness is embodied, not abstract.

STEP 4: PRACTICE PERSPECTIVE-TAKING

From this wider, steadier place, gently ask yourself one of the following questions:

- *What might I be missing when I see through only one limited lens?*
- *How might someone I trust see this situation differently?*
- *What would love require of me here?*

You're not trying to agree with another perspective—only to *imagine* it.

This stretches the mind beyond dominance into empathy, humility, hospitality, and generosity.

Often this is where the grip of certainty loosens or the flood of emotion settles—not because it's suppressed, but because it's now being held in a larger frame.

STEP 5: RETURN TO CENTER

Before moving on, ask one final question:

- *From this more centered place, what is mine to do—or not do—right now?*

The answer may be action, or restraint.

A conversation, or a pause.

Repair, or rest.

A renewed mind does not rush. It responds.

STEP 6: CLOSE IN SURRENDERED TRUST

You might close with a simple prayer or intention, like the one at the top of the chapter by St. Brendan the Navigator:

Help me to journey beyond the familiar and into the unknown.
Give me the faith to leave old ways and break fresh ground with you.
Christ of the mysteries,
I trust you to be stronger than each storm within me.
I will trust in the darkness and know
that my times, even now, are in your hand.

Then return to your day—not fixed, not finished, but a little more grounded, a little more whole, a little more capable of faith-filled and embodied love.

CHAPTER 8

resilient

Imagining Hope in a "What Doesn't Kill You Makes You Stronger" World

It's like in the great stories, Mr. Frodo. The ones that really mattered. Full of darkness and danger they were, and sometimes you didn't want to know the end. Because how could the end be happy? . . . I know now. Folk in those stories had lots of chances of turning back, only they didn't. They kept going because they were holding on to something. . . . That there's some good in this world, Mr. Frodo. And it's worth fighting for.

SAMWISE GAMGEE, *THE TWO TOWERS* FILM

Therefore we do not lose heart.

2 CORINTHIANS 4:16

"Look at you out shopping," she said. "You're so resilient, Chuck!"

I hardly had words for her. She'd been sitting in my last adult education class just days before, the very same Sunday several elders told me that the senior pastor wanted me fired from my pastoral role—and that they'd agreed to his wish.

I wasn't resilient.

I'd just emerged from three days immersed in shame. My wife didn't want to run into anyone from church at the grocery store, so I volunteered to go, praying that I'd get in and out without one of these encounters.

I wasn't resilient. I was repressing rage.

This woman's sentiment is one that's familiar to so many of us. She was saying, "You're handling this so well." In other words, she was commenting on my character at some level. She didn't say it in so many words and perhaps didn't intend it this way, but what I picked up was, *Good job stuffing it down, Chuck. No one wants your pity party. Pick yourself up and get back in the game.*

Too many people today see stoic resignation as part and parcel of good, sturdy character.

Dear reader: The word *resilience* has been hijacked.

It's been appropriated by a culture that prizes grit, grind, and endless go, go, go. It's been commandeered as a means of hustling through the hard times rather than allowing healing at the core.

These days, it's not surprising to find all sorts of examples of *performative resilience*—a curated strength that shows up in Instagram captions about "bouncing back," T-shirts emblazoned with "Keep Calm and Carry On," and saccharine sermons on overcoming the hard times or choosing joy, among other triumphal clichés. It's been shaped into a cheap imitation of Christian character—a steely exterior that traffics in self-sufficiency and not surrender.

It's the kind of faux resilience that hides our deep ache, confusing suppression with strength. This try-harder spirituality lives in the myth of control, when God invites us to hope for something so much better. It wears a mask of sufficiency while hiding weakness, the very opposite of the gospel message. The very opposite of Christlike character.

Stuffing my rage and hurt in the grocery store was my go-to response back then. I'd inherited a grit-it-out mentality. My mom grew up in Brooklyn, my dad in Queens, and in the Long Island suburb where I was raised I often felt like a misfit—a tenderhearted kid in a world of tough guys. I remember busting my knee open during a pick-up football game. Even as blood gushed from my wound, a buddy told me, "Get over it—it's just a scratch." A quiet shame loomed within during my high school and college years, whispering, "You're too soft, too emotional—toughen up if you want to fit in." I forged my mask of faux resilience in those days.

We hear that same defiant stoicism in songs—anthems that shout "What doesn't kill you makes you stronger,"[1] forgoing space for softness, sorrow, and the slow rebuild that real resilience requires. We see it in movies, where resilience is framed as brute toughness—the hero who clenches his jaw, powers through, and never sheds a tear.

But not in the 1994 film *The Shawshank Redemption*. It might have been the first movie that offered me an alternative imagination. I recall watching it for the first time in my mid-twenties, when I was stuck in self-contempt. But this film moved me. I saw that resilience could look like tenderness and trust—not just grit, but grace under pressure—a commitment to what Eugene Peterson calls "a long obedience in the same direction."[2]

Spanning almost two and a half hours, the movie conveys the slow grind of time in a place designed to break the human spirit. Shawshank State Prison is a world of concrete and conformity—a place where inmates either combust in anger or collapse into despair.

But a wrongly convicted inmate named Andy Dufresne subverts this reality.

He does not deny where he is, nor does he resign himself to it. Instead, he allows the ache to birth hope. And he fixes his eyes on something beyond those walls—a quiet beach in Zihuatanejo, Mexico; a small hotel; a boat to restore—all offering promise of a new life, fueling his resilience. That imagined future becomes for him an internal refuge, shaping how he moves through the monotony, how he treats others, and how he endures injustice. His resilience is not merely toughness or abject survival; it is imaginative fidelity to a future he has not yet seen.[3]

We see this in the best stories—the ones that echo something deep and even ancient in us. We hear the resonance in Samwise Gamgee's words from the top of the chapter: "It's like in the great stories, Mr. Frodo. The ones that really mattered. Full of darkness and danger they were, and sometimes you didn't want to know the end. Because how could the end be happy? . . . I know now. Folk in those stories had lots of chances of turning back, only they didn't. They kept going because they were holding on to something."[4]

What do we see? We see a kind of buoyancy—an inner steadiness that keeps people afloat when life's waters churn. Instead of being dragged under by overwhelm or flailing in panic, resilience lets you rise, regain breath, and find your bearings again, even when the waves are high.

Resilience, dear reader, is the fruit of a life that we've imagined thus far throughout the book—a life that is regulated, rooted, and reflective, a life that has found buoyancy even amidst the suffering. You see resilient hope in the soft faces of Samwise Gamgee and Andy Dufresne, whose eyes are drawn to something beyond the grit-it-out present, something that allows their grip to relax and their hope to expand.

You see it throughout Scripture, not least in both Hannah and Mary, the mother of Jesus. They embody a buoyant hope that rises above fear, shame, and uncertainty—an inner steadiness that keeps them from sinking beneath their circumstances. Each turns toward

God with a trusting, resilient openness, confident that something good is being birthed even before they can see it.

You hear this expansive hope in the prophets of old, like Ezekiel, who amidst valleys of dry bones looks ahead to God's promised restoration of Israel and proclaims, "They will say, 'This land that was laid waste has become like the garden of Eden'" (Ezekiel 36:35).

The kind of character-shaping resilience I long to see in myself and those I care for is nourished by two things: self-compassion and a seeing spirit.

Let's take a look at both.

Self-Compassion

How do you navigate the challenges of your life? Amidst change, do you find yourself flexible or tight? Adaptive or resistant?

Our resilience is often tested in life's most difficult moments:

- a relational rupture—a spouse's confession, a child's meltdown, the loss of a friendship—that pierces the facade and exposes the ache beneath the routine
- a surprising job loss that prompts a primal panic and insecurity
- a season of burnout that leads to vocational and personal disruption
- a quiet panic that creeps in on a sabbatical or a vacation, when the noise dies down and you're left alone with yourself for the first time in years
- a reckoning in the mirror, as you stand face-to-face with midlife questions, spiritual doubt, aging, loneliness, or regret that can no longer be numbed

- a sermon, a poem, or a song that names something so precisely you can't help but weep, without knowing why
- a confrontation with a long-unacknowledged addiction
- a failure so total and public that the false self no longer has anywhere to hide

It's often here that our old protective strategies are awakened. In the face of an unanticipated intrusion that destabilizes and disrupts, our body's survival mechanisms might lean toward anxious self-protection or numbing disconnection. Indeed, in today's culture, either grit-it-out effort or stuff-the-pain avoidance may be rewarded; they might even be seen as virtuous.

Perhaps you notice within yourself a tendency to assume this survival orientation. It may manifest within you as

- fight—a defensive-and-determined toughness
- flight—a run-from-the-problem avoidance
- fawn—a people-pleasing codependence
- find—a latch-on-to-another-for-comfort dependence
- freeze—a panicky-and-numb stuckness
- fold—an I-can't-do-this-anymore shutdown

Our bodies and brains do, indeed, have mechanisms to grind our way through or numb out. The survival mechanisms may help in the short run, but they're not fueled by hope.

What if there was another way, one that could release you from the grip of your reflexive survival responses in order to live more fully (John 10:10)? What if you were designed by a wise Creator to not merely grit it out but to grow more buoyant through your struggles?

I want you to know that it's possible to train your brain and body toward greater resilience by cultivating self-compassion and a hopeful imagination. In fact, your nervous system was designed by the Creator with this very promising reality in mind.

But like Andy in Shawshank, your circumstances might not change overnight.

When I first met Maria ten years ago, she was living in a tightly wound survival posture. Her disruption hadn't arrived with a torrent but with a slow trickle—new details seeping out about a yearslong cover-up of child sexual abuse in her denomination and church.

Back then, she tried hard not to feel any of it. She carried herself like someone who could stay objective, wise, and above the fray. But as the truth continued to surface, a quiet fury grew inside her until it finally erupted during a congregational meeting when the pastor—her family's longtime friend—confessed his role in concealing the abuse. Her angry call for accountability was met with silence, and the moderator quickly moved on.

Later, she told me she felt embarrassed by her outburst. So she buried her anger for almost two years, keeping herself in a vigilant, armored state until she finally walked into my office. She arrived exhausted and brittle, convinced that the only way to make it through was to grit her teeth and harden her heart.

In those early sessions she revealed her sense of not being safe, seen, soothed, or secure. The very thought of connecting with her emotions felt threatening. Any hint of compassion toward herself felt impossible—almost dangerous. Toughness was the only language she trusted. And yet, dutifully, she kept going to her church.

"I'm not letting them take this from me," she said. "They don't get to take my church."

But over time—so slowly she barely noticed it at first—her heart softened. She began letting herself feel small moments of tenderness for the parts of her still holding pain. A gentle hand to her heart during a panic spike. A whispered acknowledgment, "Of course this hurts," when old feelings of betrayal resurfaced.

Self-compassion didn't come naturally to her. It felt foreign, even suspicious. But it became the doorway through which she finally began to breathe again. As she learned to turn toward herself with kindness rather than contempt, something shifted. Her internal world grew less hostile. Her body settled more easily. Her reactions became less explosive and more grounded. She no longer needed toughness to survive; she was learning to trust her own tenderness as a source of buoyancy.

A decade later, she is not the same woman who first walked into my office, clenched and bracing for impact. Now she carries herself with a quiet confidence, rooted not in stoicism but in kindness toward her own wounded places. Her resilience today flows from the self-compassion she once believed she didn't deserve—and that has become, in the end, the very thing that set her free.

What is different? Well, many things changed over that time, but the core to her resilience journey was growth in self-compassion. This literally changed the state of her body and brain, a phenomenon called neuroplasticity.

Neuroplasticity, quite simply, invites us to recognize that our brains and bodies are designed to change, and change for the better.[5] You might not have noticed, but you've already used the science of neuroplasticity if you've engaged the exercises in this book! When we meet our inner experiences with the kind of openness and empathy Maria met hers with, we activate integrative circuits in the brain's middle prefrontal cortex, that region (as we've seen) responsible for regulation, attunement, emotional balance, response flexibility, and more.[6] In other words, we create the internal conditions for resilience rather than reactivity. And so our character matures—from reactive survival toward resilient love, from despair's gravity toward hope's buoyancy.

Maybe you're dug in. Maybe you feel stuck. Maybe you're weary of every disruption unleashing within you either a reactive rage or a nascent numbing. Maybe you long, like I do, to be a person who meets the suffering with greater resilience.

This begins in kindness—a kindness that you can extend to yourself, that you can receive from a dear friend, a mentor, even God. Until you're comfortable with yourself, you'll never be at ease with others, particularly during life's challenges.

Centuries ago, the Spanish reformer and mystic St. Teresa of Ávila saw the tumult in her followers and offered them this kind invitation: "Oh, souls set free by the blood of Christ! Learn to understand yourselves. Have compassion for yourselves."[7] Similarly, her contemporary in France, Bishop Francis de Sales, wrote, "Be patient with everyone, but above all with yourself. . . . Do not be disheartened by your imperfections, but always rise up with fresh courage."[8] The Christian tradition is filled with calls to a self-compassion founded on the unfathomable compassion of God.

You see, resilience—contrary to popular messaging—isn't about trying harder, but trying softer, as Christian therapist Aundi Kolber says.[9] It's about approaching yourself with a kindness that acknowledges it all—the self-sufficient strategies you've engaged, the pain you've endured, the shame you've kept under wraps. It's about allowing yourself to experience the gentle gaze of a compassionate God who meets you right where you are with a kind "Where are you?"[10]

In order to become the kind of person who bears the fruit of love, joy, peace, patience, kindness, goodness, faithfulness, gentleness, and self-control, you need to experience these in yourself. The science of neuroplasticity reminds us that self-empathy and self-compassion are prerequisites for a life of other-centered empathy and compassion. Our love of neighbor begins with love of self (see Matthew 22:39). And this is an unfolding process, not a quick fix.

By activating the integrative circuitry of your brain, you are galvanizing a full-brained, full-bodied, wholehearted, God-created design system for the sake of your long-term transformation.

This, of course, reminds us again of the futility of performative change. When we attempt to rush character change, we undermine the very neurobiological processes necessary for long-term transformation. We may attempt cosmetic change with a quick word of repentance and a few new behaviors, but we're likely operating out of a survival orientation. This is a pick-yourself-up-by-your-bootstraps-and-soldier-on form of faux resilience, and though it's popular today, it's not at all the path to real change.

While self-compassion is the first whole-brained-and-bodied path to real resilience, there is also a second track. And this one illuminates why we love the old stories—the clear-eyed vision of an Andy Dufresne or a Sam Gamgee, and the hearty hope of Hannah and Mary.

A Seeing Spirit

When our bodies and brains are locked in a survival orientation, we can't change. We'll fight it. We might talk about the therapy we're doing or the sabbatical we're taking or the books we're reading, but our nervous systems will simply not allow for deep transformation. This is why it's so critical to begin by creating the conditions for change.

Once we've learned to meet our present state with self-compassion—neither fighting it nor fleeing its reality—we can imagine our way into a hopeful future. Like Andy in *The Shawshank Redemption*, we can long, even ache, for our Zihuatanejo.

In the months after my emergency surgery and sepsis scare, which I now see was brought on by the trauma and suppression I experienced after being fired from my pastoral role, I began to consider a whole-brained-and-whole-bodied path forward for my own healing. In those early days, I sifted through the varied resources on the science of brain change, and soon I noticed a theme. Practitioners of deep change would continually ask, *Who do you long to be?* Hopeful imagination, I discovered, is core to real resilience and healing.[11] And it's not surprising, through a Christian lens, that nurturing hope might be crucial to deep change.

I recall a skeptical season when I'd been practicing neural retraining, which led me to create a catchphrase that summarized the type of person I wanted to be.[12] I'd never done anything like this, and I'm wary of anything that seems like a form of bypassing, particularly through the power of positive thinking. But I went along with the training, creating a hopeful axiom—"I am calm and present with energy and joy."

Along with a hopeful mantra, neural retraining encourages people to add hand gestures to concretize the practice, which I did, albeit self-consciously at first. I'd place my left hand on my heart to symbolize calm. I'd open my hands with palms up to represent presence. I'd raise my hands a little higher to signify energy. And place both of my hands over each other on my chest to embody joy.

I'd awake each morning envisioning a future self who embodied these realities. I'd imagine sitting with clients and students in my office, teaching my classes, speaking at a conference, engaging my wife and kids—all from a place of *calm*, *presence*, *energy*, and *joy*. Each word symbolized my intention to make a fundamental shift—from a chaotic life to a calm one, from preoccupation to presence, from exhausting patterns to wholehearted energy, from judgmental to joyful. I was practicing the neurobiology of character change.

And I was nurturing a hopeful imagination, not unlike what the prophets of old did, those who saw through current circumstances and calamities into a new future. (See, for example, Isaiah 65:17-19 and Revelation 21:3-5.)

But as I continued learning, I adopted another critical practice once I discovered that the real neurological punch is not merely in the words or gestures, but in the felt experience of each.[13] In other words, it wasn't enough to say or symbolize the words *calm and present with energy and joy*. It was important to feel and embody the reality—to give my whole being the lived experience of real calm, presence, energy, and joy.

Open to continued growth, I deepened my embodied practice. I'd often begin by finding my way to a quiet place, with my eyes closed and my left hand over my heart, breathing gently—four seconds in, holding for seven, exhaling for eight. I'd notice any survival energy in me—usually a bit of fight, flight, or fawn—and relax into my body, sensing a growing connection within. With the gestures and words *calm*, *present*, *energy*, and *joy*, I'd allow myself to feel and embody each. At first, it felt a little forced, even manufactured. But in a matter of days, I couldn't wait to wake up to my practice, even to repeat it several times throughout the day. My body and brain were learning. After years of living with my fuel tank in the red, I was finding surprising reserves and growing resilience.

When we imagine our future selves with vivid detail and with authentic emotional engagement, we activate the same neural pathways that would be involved if we were actually living that future. What's stunning is your brain doesn't fully distinguish between what is vividly imagined and what is real. This means that repeated mental rehearsal of a hopeful, embodied future can begin to rewire neural circuits—strengthening pathways associated with connection, calm, joy, presence, energy, attunement, and more.

Emotion is the catalyst.

As we combine a positive affect with focused attention, we signal the brain: *This matters. Reinforce this.* Your brain's prefrontal cortex engages to imagine possibility, your limbic system contributes the felt meaning, and your default mode network helps you envision a hopeful future. By consistently practicing who we long to become, we lay down the neural scaffolding of that future self—long before it fully arrives.

Today, more than a decade and a half after I began engaging this work, I feel much more like that future self I envisioned than the guy stuck in chaos, preoccupation, exhaustion, and judgment. That's not to say he's gone. I still have memories of those old prison walls, and sometimes I live as if I'm still there. I lived in Storm and Fog for a long, long time—and my body remembers. However, my body also reminds me every day that I'm more healthy and whole in my mid-fifties than I was in my early forties.

Character transformation begins in safety, self-compassion, and connection—when our brains and bodies experience the spiritual, psychological, and physiological conditions necessary for resilience.

But it is nurtured in hope, as our deepest longings to become a "new creation" (2 Corinthians 5:17) are intentionally engaged with an earnest hope for maturation. If you've been engaging not just the words but the practices of this book, then you, too, are cultivating this earnest hope—and transformative change.

Earnest Hope

The apostle James writes, "Let perseverance finish its work so that you may be mature [*teleios*] and complete, not lacking anything" (James 1:4). The perseverance James speaks of is not white-knuckled willpower but a resiliency that grows in our steadfast commitment to staying in the struggle and not avoiding it. It's a resilience that resists futile fatalism or naive idealism.

And I'm suggesting that this hopeful work is so much better than our cherished habits of numbing, avoiding, chasing, clinging, and more.

Andy Dufresne imagined himself in Zihuatanejo amidst a decades-long exile. I picture him mentally rehearsing that future day when the sun wouldn't be impeded by concrete walls and steel bars, when the gentle breeze coming off the ocean would refresh him in body and soul. His hopeful imagination borrows from the saints of old, prophets who offered an exhilarating possibility amidst harrowing circumstances, even bewildering exile. Isaiah wrote:

> This is what the Lord says—
>   he who made a way through the sea,
>   a path through the mighty waters,
> who drew out the chariots and horses,
>   the army and reinforcements together,

and they lay there, never to rise again,
    extinguished, snuffed out like a wick:
"Forget the former things;
    do not dwell on the past.
See, I am doing a new thing!
    Now it springs up; do you not perceive it?
I am making a way in the wilderness
    and streams in the wasteland."

ISAIAH 43:16-19

Indeed, in the dark we find ourselves squinting, hoping to see just a glimpse of the way God is making for us. The prophets promised no Hollywood ending. But they did awaken—in body and soul—the hope of a day when freedom would reign.

Martin Luther King Jr. inspired the same hopeful imagination one summer day in 1963, amidst a throng of onlookers longing for their cherished liberation:

> I have a dream that one day on the red hills of Georgia, the sons of former slaves and the sons of former slave owners will be able to sit down together at the table of brotherhood. . . .
>
> I have a dream that my four little children will one day live in a nation where they will not be judged by the color of their skin but by the content of their character. I have a dream today. . . .
>
> I have a dream that one day every valley shall be exalted, every hill and mountain shall be made low, the rough places will be made plain, and the crooked places will be made straight, and the glory of the Lord shall be revealed, and all flesh shall see it together.[14]

King didn't anticipate what would happen almost five years later when he'd be murdered by the bullet of an assassin. We never know what the future may hold, or how short or long our lives might be. There isn't a promised timetable, although Scripture and history reveal how lengthy the wait for healing often is. But we are invited to hold in our bodies and imaginations the possibility of shalom—even rehearsing it in the here and now.

I recall days when I felt like nothing I did mattered or helped, days when I thought I'd feel broken forever. Yet amidst what seemed like unchanging realities around me, there was something hopeful about reengaging the work within. While I couldn't control things around me, I could curate a fresh experience within, laying down the new, neural scaffolding for the future self I was building. I awakened to my practices each day, not with a posture of dogged determination but with eager expectation. Indeed, it's God's grace that changes us—but we're invited to cooperate and participate, even through an engagement of our God-created bodies and brains.

Paul says, "Therefore, if anyone is in Christ, the new creation has come: The old has gone, the new is here!" (2 Corinthians 5:17). And while Paul knew all too well that his own circumstances were often frustrating, even dire at times, he spoke to the inner reality of his Spirit-born self. The tug of the old self still existed, with its propensity to shame and fear, with its insistence on law and self-reliance. But he was challenging the Corinthian church to live into the reality of the new reconciled, empowered, and enlivened self within, reoriented toward love, grace, and freedom. Perhaps that challenge is for you and me too.

Cultivating hope catalyzes character change.

Who do you long to be? How do you long to live?

And how might small changes you make today shape the person you are becoming?

And so, dear friends,

May you come to know resilience
not as a clenched jaw or a steeled spine,
but as the quiet courage to stay present to what is—
with a heart still open to what could be.

May you come to know hope
not as a pie-in-the-sky fantasy
but as a longing for shalom
at the depths of your being and for the heart of the world.

And when the path is long and the exile lingers,
may you not harden, but soften.
Knowing that in the unseen rewiring of your brain and being,
Christ forms in you a future.

"See, I am doing a new thing!
Now it springs up; do you not perceive it?
I am making a way in the wilderness
and streams in the wasteland."

RESOURCES

- Aundi Kolber, *Try Softer: A Fresh Approach to Move Us out of Anxiety, Stress, and Survival Mode—and into a Life of Connection and Joy*
- Jeffrey M. Schwartz and Sharon Begley, *The Mind and the Brain: Neuroplasticity and the Power of Mental Force*
- Daniel J. Siegel, *Mindsight: The New Science of Personal Transformation*
- N. T. Wright, *Surprised by Hope: Rethinking Heaven, the Resurrection, and the Mission of the Church*

REFLECTION

1. How have you heard or experienced the word *resilience* being used by friends, the church, or contemporary culture? What impact has that had on you, even on your way of living and being?
2. Consider the first aspect of resilience—self-compassion. How have you experienced self-compassion in your own life? How might you begin to see self-compassion as a crucial part of your own change process?
3. Think about the second aspect of resilience—a seeing spirit. How does it feel to consider this pathway and practice to nurture hope? If you tend to be future-oriented and naively hopeful, how might this pathway invite you to a more real and grounded hope? If you tend to be more past-oriented or even fatalistic, how might this stretch you into imagining who you long to become?
4. What parts of you tend to get stuck in one or more of the six F's?

   fight—a defensive-and-determined toughness

   flight—a run-from-the-problem avoidance

   fawn—a people-pleasing codependence

find—a latch-on-to-another-for-comfort dependence

freeze—a panicky-and-numb stuckness

fold—an I-can't-do-this-anymore shutdown

How might you approach yourself with compassion as you recognize your propensity to one or more of these reactions? What might it be like to live beyond this reality?

5. Imagine yourself in ten years through the same hopeful lens of the prophets of old, who often began their long descriptions with the word "Behold." Write your own description of your future self—"Behold, this is who [your name] is becoming, reflected by . . ." With this prompt, describe the kinds of soul-and-body changes you long to see.

PRACTICE
Cultivating Resilience for the Sake of Character Change

A Self-Compassion Practice

STEP 1: ARRIVE IN YOUR BODY

- Sit or stand comfortably.
- Let your breath lengthen just a bit—nothing forced, simply steady.
- Feel the weight of your body, the ground beneath you.

STEP 2: PLACE A HAND ON YOUR HEART OR BELLY

This is a cue of warmth and presence.

Let your system know: *I'm here. The Spirit is here.*

STEP 3: GREET THE PARTS THAT ARE PRESENT

Imagine standing at the doorway of your inner home as the day begins.

One by one, notice which parts are awake and lingering nearby.

- If there is a weary part:
  Good morning, tired one. I see how much you've carried.
  Offer it a soft nod of compassion.
- If a wounded part is stirring:
  Hello, tender one. You don't need to hide. I'll be gentle with you today.
- If a wandering or distracted part is already moving fast:
  Hi there, restless one. You're welcome too. You don't have to figure everything out right now.
- If a protective part stands guard:
  Thank you for watching over me. You've helped me survive. You can soften if you want to, or stay close if you need.

STEP 4: LET EACH PART BE EXACTLY AS IT IS

No fixing.

No pushing away.

Just presence.

As each part appears, meet it with the three postures of compassion: curiosity, warmth, and nonjudgment.

STEP 5: CLOSE WITH A COLLECTIVE BLESSING

Gently say:

May you all feel welcome today.

And may you feel embraced, even by God's Spirit.

Here, I no longer need to fight or flee, fawn or find, freeze or fold.

Here, I'm safely held in love.

Here, I can expand, in buoyant hope, knowing I'm free.

Take one more slow breath.

Step into the day accompanied, not alone.

A Seeing Spirit Practice

STEP 1: SELECT A PHRASE OR SENTENCE THAT REFLECTS THE VISION OF WHO YOU LONG TO BECOME

This hopeful maxim reflects your imagination of a future self who embodies the characteristics you hope to become. Mine was "I am calm and present with energy and joy." Each word symbolized my intention to shift from a chaotic life to calm, from preoccupied to present, from exhausted to energetic, from judgy to joyful.

What would your aspirational sentence be?

STEP 2: COME UP WITH HAND GESTURES TO COUPLE WITH EACH WORD

Such gestures will help you reinforce the vision you set for yourself. For me, "calm" was represented by a hand on my chest; I opened my hands in front of me for "present"; I opened and raised my hands higher when saying, "energy"; and I placed one hand on top of the other on my chest as I said "joy."

STEP 3: ALLOW YOURSELF TIME TO REALLY FEEL AND EMBODY THE REALITY

Give your whole being the lived experience of real calm, presence, energy, and joy.[15] To do this, find a quiet space. You might engage earlier practices that cultivate feelings of being safe, seen, soothed, and secure. When you're ready, consider the following:

- Take some time to imagine this future you—feel in your body what it's like to be [fill in the blank]. I imagined myself being *calm, present, energetic, and joyful*.
- Linger here, reflecting on each embodied reality. Really feel *calm*. Really feel *presence*. Really feel *energy*. Really feel *joy*. Feel each

word, in your heart, in your whole body. Imagine what it would be like to experience the fullness of each.

- Fill your lungs with air, inhaling goodness, Eden's ancient echo arising in your body even now. Feel what it's like to flourish within. Linger here. See the smile of your future self. Imagine God's smile in whatever way feels natural or nourishing to your soul. (I like to imagine the joy of God greeting me like the prodigal son in Luke 15, a story in which the father has attributes of both mother and father as he runs to and embraces his child.)

STEP 4: BRING THIS NEW YOU INTO A CONCRETE SITUATION THROUGH YOUR IMAGINATION

Now, imagine bringing this *you*—calm, present, energetic, joyful—into a concrete moment of your everyday life. Picture yourself walking into your home at the end of the day, sitting down at your desk, or entering a conversation that usually carries some tension. Notice what happens in your body as you do. Does your chest tighten? Does your breath shorten? Does an old familiar pull toward urgency, self-protection, or self-judgment arise?

Rather than correcting or overriding these responses, simply stay with them. Breathe slowly and gently. Let this imagined future self remain present *with* the activation rather than trying to escape it. You might quietly remind yourself: *I am safe right now. I don't need to rush. I can stay.* Notice how calm, presence, energy, or joy (or whatever realities you envision) can coexist with difficulty—not as perfection, but as resilient capacity.

Linger here for a few moments. Let your body learn that this way of being is not just possible in stillness, but it is available—again and again—in the midst of real life.

CHAPTER 9

relational

Embodying Love Amidst Anxious and Avoidant Systems

There is a false form of honesty that suggests that nothing should remain hidden and that everything should be said, expressed and communicated. This honesty can be very harmful, and if it does not harm, it at least makes the relationship flat, superficial, empty and often very boring.

HENRI NOUWEN

Abide in Me, and I in you. As the branch cannot bear fruit of itself, unless it abides in the vine, neither can you, unless you abide in Me. I am the vine, you are the branches. He who abides in Me, and I in him, bears much fruit; for without Me you can do nothing. If anyone does not abide in Me, he is cast out as a branch and is withered.

JOHN 15:4-6, NKJV

Sometimes my longing to love gets entangled with my need to please. And I'm not sure if I'm caring well or currying favor.

It happened one Saturday morning when I received a message through a social media platform.

"If you really cared," a man had written, "you'd post more about what's happening in our politics right now."

I was jolted by the message, and my body immediately tightened—my chest constricted; my breathing became shallow. Recent days had been filled with a barrage of news stories, each more unnerving than the last. There was a palpable sense of urgency in the air to speak against injustice. Now I felt pulled to say something merely to relieve the acute stress I felt.

I was feeling the stormy swirl of it all in my body, but I was also trying to stay attuned to my wife, and to my daughters, then in high school and asking their own hard questions about our fraught politics. On top of that, I was tending to my clients, some of whom were significantly triggered by the unfolding events. And then there were my students, with their own inner storms. A colleague and I were working on convening a time of lament and prayer for them.

And still, I felt convicted by the sharp message I received. A sense of guilt started growing in me, so strong so that I began crafting a post for social media. It was a Saturday morning, and I'd written and re-written several versions before my wife and daughters woke up. By then, my agitation was noticeable to them and to me.

I tried to put the attempt aside, but my mind played with words throughout the day, stealing attention from my family. I did post something, but I also felt uneasy, like I'd forced it. I snuck online to check on the post a few times, only to see comments growing—some scathing. Finally, one of my daughters asked, "Why are you being like this today?" It was well after dinner at that point, our day disrupted by my lack of presence.

We're often pulled by relational forces, some so strong that we feel untethered, prompting reaction rather than reflection. Thankfully, I was caught in a temporary storm, and soon enough I was able to find my ground again—and words to own the hurt I'd caused my family. But this relational energy can shape a life of rootlessness, where we feel tossed in the wind rather than grounded in who we're becoming. And it can shape the way we love, disposing us to a life of pleasing and performance, compromising our capacity for authentic compassion and wholehearted affection.

Performative Compassion

That stressful Saturday ended with a question that arose as I lay down to sleep: What does it mean to love?

It's a complicated question, isn't it? It's particularly complex in a day when our relationships aren't simply local and familial but are extended by tethers of digital connection, even across the globe.

Despite the accusatory tone of the message I received, I'd like to think that the person who wrote it really longed to know, "Chuck, what does it mean for you to love?"

I'd like to believe that he'd be open to an unhurried conversation about what it means to care well in an anxious age, and that I'd be calm enough to have it. But I wasn't calm when I posted my comment. I was chaotically storming within, frantically forming words in my head until I could type them out and hit "post," pining for a dopamine-charged sense of release.

I had hoped my carefully crafted words would convey a sense of authentic conviction and compassion, but the execution was ultimately performative. Additionally, my anxious obsessing had deprived my family of love and attunement. In the end, I'd spent the better part of a Saturday in an exhausting exercise of virtue signaling.

The origins of the term *virtue signaling* are often attributed to a 2015 *Spectator* essay by journalist James Bartholomew, who described a growing trend of public moral posturing—expressing virtuous opinions not to effect change but to bolster one's image.[1]

Though the concept draws from prior psychological theories of social signaling, its modern usage highlights a shift in empathy from genuine presence to performance, from *real* compassion to *being seen* as compassionate.

Performative compassion.

And while it's easy to render a quick judgment of someone who reacts in this way, it may be an indicator of a deeper relational orientation—or what some might call poor differentiation.

I first learned about differentiation through the lens of Murray Bowen's family systems theory when I was training as a therapist.[2] As is the case with so much of what's learned in this kind of intensive training, I immediately saw my own family of origin reflected in the concepts.

Differentiation is the ability to maintain a strong sense of self while remaining meaningfully connected to others. But I grew up in a poorly differentiated family, where my sense of self was fused to my mother's sense of self. Our emotional enmeshment compromised my capacity to attune to my unique needs and desires, instead orienting me around external expectations—like my mother's affection or approval. It established relational patterns that I've had to disrupt and dismantle over many years. But I'm clearly not immune to being pulled back into the dynamic.

When we're undifferentiated, boundaries between ourselves and others become blurred. We mistake fusion for connection and sacrifice authenticity for approval. In other words, I lose "me" in caring for you. And that's what happened on that anxious Saturday after I received the message.

If I'd been differentiated in a healthy way, I would have been "rooted and grounded in love" (Ephesians 3:17, NKJV), which is to say, anchored in a connected sense of myself. I would have felt no need to seek outside what was already mine: the inviolable inheritance of worth, belonging, and purpose as God's beloved that Christ longs to give to all people.[3] With healthy differentiation, I would have been able to

- discern a sense of real inner conviction from the need for validation;
- act out of my core values, rather than responding to the disappointments and demands of others;
- remain connected to my own internal experience and my family's need for my presence, and even to that critic's needs; and
- love in a way that was pure and whole.

This is how God created us. You and I were designed in the image of the Trinity—God's image bearers created in and for relationship (Genesis 1–2). It was the twisted lies of the serpent, however, that propelled humanity into an unhealthy externalization (Genesis 3). Adam and Eve snatched what they thought would give them joy and a sense of empowerment, and we've been grasping ever since. Recognizing my own tendency to look in the wrong places for validation and belonging, I often ask myself, *How am I chasing worth, belonging, or purpose? And how does this compromise my capacity to love well?*

Differentiation and Love

To understand the stormy swirl that arises within us, we need to talk more about differentiation.

Differentiation is the fruit of maturity, manifesting in a secure self and a spacious presence for others. Differentiation, I'd contend, fulfills the law of love articulated by Jesus when he said, "'Love the Lord your God with all your heart and with all your soul and with all your mind.' This is the first and greatest commandment. And the second is like it: 'Love your neighbor as yourself.' All the Law and the Prophets hang on these two commandments" (Matthew 22:37-40). And this is at the heart of character formation.

Without differentiation, we're prone to fall into one of two ditches: We either become enmeshed or detached. Both compromise our capacity to authentically love and be loved, ultimately shaping our character around either fusion or flight.

In enmeshment, we lose ourselves in others' emotions, expectations, or approval. This is what happened to me when I was confronted by the social media message. My locus of control shifted from a grounded, stable internal sense of myself to a chaotic, muddled, externalized sense of myself, activating a fawning pattern my body knew from childhood. Just as we've seen in prior chapters, I shifted from connection to survival.

And my thought patterns and relational behaviors followed. I was consumed all day by sensing someone's disappointment in me. I was lost in my head, trying to form the right language for what I considered to be an appropriately worded and compassionate social media post.

Consider the everyday ways this dynamic shows up:

- A woman anxiously monitors her boyfriend's moods, changing her opinions and silencing her needs to maintain his affection, fearing that disagreement could mean abandonment.

- A parent overidentifies with their child's success, feeling personal failure when the child struggles and intruding by attempting to control outcomes rather than supporting growth.
- A friend who can't say no constantly reshuffles her life to accommodate others' expectations; then quietly resents it while feeling guilty for setting boundaries.
- A social media influencer performs outrage or empathy, not from grounded conviction, but to maintain relevance, approval, or belonging within a particular ideological tribe.
- A leader mirrors the anxiety of the system, reacting impulsively to conflict or pressure rather than remaining a calm, principled presence who can contain and guide others through difficulty.

The reality is, each of us likely has some sort of connection to this phenomenon, even if it hasn't been a long-term pattern.

The second ditch we can fall into is detachment, which leads us to withdraw inwardly to preserve a fragile sense of self. Here, the locus of control shifts from a grounded, stable internal sense of self to a rigid, self-protected internal sense of self. This might show up as avoidance, emotional numbing, or strict boundaries. In detachment, we protect ourselves from the vulnerability of connection by disengaging, but this also isolates us and stunts relational depth.

If I learned fusion with my mother, I learned detachment in relationship with my father. I watched my dad retreat amidst anxiety, usually when conflict would arise with my mom. I often found myself in internal conflict—should I attune to my mother's needs or join my father in disconnection? Those closest to me have likely seen this pattern play out: Will Chuck stay connected and appease or isolate and avoid?

Consider the everyday ways this dynamic shows up:

- A husband shuts down during conflict, retreating into silence or busyness rather than risking emotional exposure, believing that self-protection is safer than connection.
- A leader intellectualizes every conversation, avoiding emotional depth by staying in the realm of abstract ideas, masking fear of intimacy with polished distance.
- A teacher keeps rigid boundaries, not to model health, but to avoid being impacted, subtly withholding empathy out of fear that closeness will demand too much.
- A friend avoids offering support during another's grief, excusing his absence with logic or scheduling conflicts, when in truth, he fears being overwhelmed by emotion.
- An adult child limits contact with his aging parents, not to maintain healthy boundaries, but because unresolved pain makes authentic connection feel intolerable.

Ultimately, fusion and detachment are two ways of managing anxiety.

Fusion says, "I'll merge with you so I don't have to feel the terror of disconnection," while detachment says, "I'll withdraw from you so I don't have to feel the threat of losing myself." Both are strategies rooted in fear—one of abandonment, the other of engulfment. And as we've learned, when we're stuck in an anxious survival orientation, it's almost impossible to connect, meaning our capacity to love is compromised.

True character formation invites us beyond these anxious extremes, cultivating a "rooted and grounded" self that can remain present in the tensions of love without fusing or fleeing.

Wired for Connection

Our relational patterns testify to what we've learned over the course of a lifetime about safety, trust, connection, survival, vulnerability, even integrity. And these patterns reveal what our brains and bodies have indexed as normal and true over time. This is why it's often so hard to see meaningful change in a leader confronted for harmful patterns of relating.

Over the years, I've been invited to consult within a wide array of systems—churches, nonprofits, small businesses, educational spaces, tech start-ups, and more. Often, I find myself in nervous *systems*—not the intricate web of nerves, brain structures, and electrical signals within the body—but the kinds of nervous systems between people.

I look around the room, wondering about each person, uniquely formed by the faces, voices, and bodies they grew up around. Each of them shaped in a particular pattern of relating. Each of them likely doing what their body has always known to do to connect and to survive. I often pay close attention to the leader or leaders, watching how they engage and interact.

Our brains are wired for connection, but undifferentiated leaders—those who either anxiously merge or rigidly detach—create emotional instability in those around them. And those within the system respond in the ways they've learned from their own families and backgrounds.

Years ago, I consulted for a large organization, led by an anxious and controlling leader. Scanning the room, my eyes landed on an older woman, likely twice the age of the leader. She sat in the back, arms folded, a vacant look on her face. During one-on-one interviews about a week later, I asked her what was happening for her during that gathering.

"I don't get it, Chuck. . . . I could be his mother, but when he's up there, it feels like I'm being scolded by my father," she told me.

"I saw you sitting there, looking distant," I said. "Where do you go in times like that?"

"I'm a little girl again, isolating in my room to avoid my father," she said. "Anything not to feel the anxiety."

We learn a lot about what's happening within us when we begin to get curious about what we feel or how we respond in relationships, groups, and systems. When an old anxiety is activated within us, we may find ourselves regressing to an earlier age, perhaps even without our conscious awareness that it's occurring.

Differentiation, then, is not merely a psychological skill—it is a nervous system capacity. When we enter a room, our bodies don't just walk in—they tune in. The human nervous system is exquisitely relational. Through what neuroscientists call mirror neurons, we unconsciously attune to the facial expressions, tone of voice, body posture, and emotional energy of those around us. This resonance happens beneath our conscious awareness: hearts begin to beat in rhythm, nervous systems begin to synchronize, emotions become shared. In short, we become like those we're with.

This is the beauty and the burden of being wired for connection. In its most life-giving form, it means that calm begets calm, safety fosters safety, and joy invites joy. A grounded, differentiated presence can serve as a kind of relational tuning fork, helping others attune to something steadier, clearer, more hopeful. But when a leader is dysregulated—overwhelmed by anxiety, seeking the approval of others, or disengaged in stoic detachment—those around them pick up that frequency, often without even realizing it.

In John 8, Jesus stands at the center of a simmering, shaming spectacle. The religious leaders drag a woman before him, weaponizing both her body and the law in an attempt to trap him. The crowd hums with moral certainty, demanding the woman be stoned to death, and yet Jesus refuses to be hurried by their urgency. He stoops. He writes in the dust. And he creates pause in a moment of intensity and escalation. Rather than matching accusation with counteraccusation, he calmly exposes the shared condition of sin—"Let any one of you who is without sin be the first to throw a stone" (verse 7). One by one, the accusers leave. Only then does he turn toward the woman, not to condemn her, but to restore agency and dignity. "Neither do I condemn you," Jesus declares. "Go now and leave your life of sin" (verse 11). Here, Jesus embodies differentiated leadership—grounded, non-anxious, unwilling to collude with shame or violence, yet unwavering in truth. And his words "Leave your life of sin" aren't meant to simply correct behavior—from a place of security, he invites her to leave behind a life of survival and enter into the joy of a life of secure love.

As Jesus models, to be differentiated is to be a nervous system in regulation even amidst the storm of dysregulation. It is the ability to stay rooted, without becoming fused with the chaos or withdrawing into isolation. It is the capacity to hold space for others, without collapsing into their anxiety or defensiveness. It is the gift of being that relational tuning fork, where security begets security, hope begets hope, joy begets joy.

Pete and Geri Scazzero, founders of Emotionally Healthy Discipleship, describe what they call the Ladder of Integrity—a pathway for remaining connected without losing oneself—all for the sake of loving others well.[4] Rather than collapsing into reactivity or withdrawing into silence when provoked, the ladder invites us first to turn inward: to notice our triggers, name what we are feeling, and discern which core values or wounds are being stirred. We've been practicing these skills throughout this book. From that grounded awareness, we can then move outward with clarity and courage—speaking honestly, setting appropriate limits, and seeking deeper understanding rather than blame. Integrity, in this sense, is not about moral perfection but the steady integration of inner life and outer response. When leaders cultivate this kind of presence, they become stabilizing forces in anxious systems—calm without being cold, compassionate without being compliant. In a fragmented world, such differentiated love is both rare and profoundly transformative.

When we cultivate this kind of presence, we become safe harbors—people whose nervous systems don't just mirror, but regulate. In families, classrooms, churches, and workplaces, it's often not the smartest or most strategic voice that creates change, but the calmest. This calm is not passivity or performance—it's the fruit of inner integration. And in a world teeming with relational complexity, this kind of grounding and loving presence is desperately needed.

The Ground from Which Empathy Grows

When we feel safe in our own bodies and secure in our relationships, something remarkable becomes possible: empathy. Not the strained, self-sacrificing version that depletes us, but an authentic empathy, emerging from a core of integrity. Our movement toward another flows from our heart, allowing us to love another without losing our center. Here, character is embodied in loving and whole relationship.

Empathy is a contemporary name for what Christians have long recognized as central to love—a deep, embodied concern that flows from the core of our being, not from duty or performance. This empathy is made visible in the incarnational love of Jesus, whose care for others rose from the very center of his compassionate heart rather than from obligation or social approval.

The New Testament Greek word *splanchnizomai* captures this beautifully. It means to be moved in your inward parts—your belly, your bowels, your womb—the ancient seat of empathy. When the Gospels tell us Jesus was "moved with compassion," it's *splanchnizomai* (see Matthew 9:36; Matthew 14:14; Luke 7:13). It reflects the ache in Jesus' gut when he sees the suffering, the scattered, the shamed. It's not pity from a distance. It's a visceral knowing, a felt resonance that moves him toward others in love.[5]

This is biblical empathy. Not self-erasure, not sentimentalism, but embodied attunement. An attunement that begins in the brain's resonance circuitry, is communicated through the body, and is aimed toward healing action. It reflects a God who not only sees, but feels—who enters into our story viscerally, in the flesh. True empathy, in the biblical sense, is true embodiment.

Today, neuroscientists and psychologists speak of empathy in three consecutive movements. Cognitive empathy is our ability to understand what another person is thinking or feeling; to see the world through their eyes. Emotional empathy moves deeper, activating our resonance circuitry within and allowing us to feel with them, resonating with their sorrow or joy. And empathic concern takes us further still, propelling us into compassionate action—not out of guilt or pressure, but out of true presence and care. These movements reflect the progression of incarnational love.

But empathy is under fire today.[6]

Some critique empathy as indulgent or manipulative, even calling it dangerous or sinful. What they're reacting to, I believe, is not true empathy, but undifferentiated empathy—empathy that lacks boundaries, discernment, and grounding in one's true self. When empathy becomes reactive or performative, when it erases the self in the process of caring for the other, it can indeed become distorted. But that is not the fault of empathy itself—it's the failure to embody it well.[7]

Critics also worry that empathy simply accepts people as they are, softening moral clarity and excusing what should be confronted. But true empathy does not collude with harm or baptize destructive behavior. It draws near without surrendering truth. It listens deeply enough to understand the fears, wounds, and survival patterns beneath the surface, and then—grounded and differentiated—it invites a person toward something freer and more whole. Empathy, rightly embodied, does not lower the bar of transformation; it makes transformation possible.

It's true—in a world addicted to optics and applause, empathy is often not an expression of love but of anxiety. It becomes performative—more about appearing to care than actually caring. It emerges not from the holy depths of the human heart, but from our fragile ego, our need to belong, to please, to be worthy, to forge some sense of purpose. This kind of empathy doesn't nourish; it exhausts, ultimately leading to empathy fatigue.[8]

This invites us to explore how we care, even the cost of our care.

Pondering over Performance

Years ago through that episode with the social media critic, I learned that I was still capable of living an undifferentiated life, which threatened my capacity to love well. That's not to say that I was incapable of love—indeed, much of the work I'd done in the years prior involved growing in my ability to care well for others. Yet, the old neural patterns hadn't fully died. I'd rehearsed them over time, and they had shaped my character. Now I was pulled to perform virtue, once again.

Dear readers, the kind of character change we've envisioned takes a lifetime. You are not minute rice. You are not microwavable popcorn. No, God's work within is slow, the ripening a process that takes longer than we'd like and that invites the renewal of our whole selves.

But there's a danger too: We need to guard against merely performing this ripening process. If narcissism is evolving in our culture, then one of its most recent modifications is the tendency to perform rather than embody vulnerability, emotional processing, spiritual growth, and even transformation. Perhaps we need to learn the slow wisdom of Mary, who witnessed all the mysterious events surrounding Jesus' birth and "treasured up all these things, pondering them in her heart" (Luke 2:19, ESV).

Years before the advent of social media, Henri Nouwen offered a prophetic insight into our current performative predicament:

> There is a false form of honesty that suggests that nothing should remain hidden and that everything should be said, expressed and communicated. This honesty can be very harmful, and if it does not harm, it at least makes the

> relationship flat, superficial, empty and often very boring. When we try to shake off our loneliness by creating a milieu without limiting boundaries, we may become entangled in a stagnating closeness. It is our vocation to prevent the harmful exposure of our inner sanctuary, not only for our own protection but also as a service to our fellow human beings with whom we want to enter in a creative communion.[9]

Nouwen's warning feels almost eerily prescient in an age in which vulnerability itself has become currency. In a hypertherapeutic culture, we are encouraged to narrate our wounds in real time, to externalize every emotion, to confuse disclosure with depth. But when confession is driven by anxiety rather than groundedness, it can become fauxnerability—an exposure that seeks relief, validation, or even control rather than real connection. Instead of deepening relationships, this kind of compulsive honesty can flatten them, turning intimacy into performance and self-awareness into self-display. What masquerades as courage may in fact be another strategy to manage loneliness or secure belonging, revealing not integration but urgency.

Decades ago, I prayed for a day when resources on emotional and spiritual health would be abundant—but I didn't anticipate how easily abundance could morph into commodification. What was meant to deepen us sometimes became another arena for self-curation. We mastered the language of attachment styles and Enneagram numbers, yet often neglected the cultivation of character. My question now is: Are we becoming a more loving, joyful, peaceful, patient, kind, good, faithful, gentle, and self-controlled people? These tools are good if, indeed, they are cultivating maturity.

But perhaps most poignant for our ripening and maturation is Nouwen's call to cultivate an "inner sanctuary"—where we can ponder, as Mary did, and then speak from a place of integrity and authenticity. This can be a place where our loves are re-shaped, where our hearts are re-formed, where our character is—in time—transformed. It's the place from which can spring the person we were intended to become all along.

This inner sanctuary is not withdrawal from the world but the deep wellspring of life (Proverbs 4:23). It is a safe refuge within—our inner "home"—where anxious striving comes to rest, where our fragmented parts are gathered, and where, like branches abiding in the vine (John 15:4–5), we remain connected to the one who animates our loving.

And from this hidden place—slowly, imperceptibly at times—character ripens. Not as spectacle, but as substance. Not as branding, but as being. In a culture of exposure and urgency, cultivating this holy inner sanctuary becomes an act of resistance and trust. It is where we are formed in secret so that, when we step into the light, what shines forth is not performance, but presence.

Dear friends, this is the work of a lifetime. It is a call to love, a call desperately needed for such a time as this.

And so:

May you resist the pull to perform love
and instead become love—slow, steady, rooted.

May the winds of opinion not unmoor you,
nor the ache of disconnection drive you to abandon your truest self.

When the world demands urgency,
may you choose presence.
When it seduces you with approval,
may you return to your inner sanctuary.

May you feel again the pulse of divine compassion,
not as pressure but as presence,
not as performance but as participation
in the slow work of becoming.

May the voice of Jesus—"Abide in me"—
settle like balm in your bones.
May it call you back when you drift,
anchor you when you waver,
and root you in love when everything feels scattered.

And when love gets tangled up in pleasing,
when empathy feels like erasure,
may you pause—breathe—and return.
To the ground beneath your feet.
To the inner sanctuary that holds you safe and secure.
To the love that never asked for your performance,
only your presence.

Abide there.
Remain there.
Grow there.
And from that rooted place,
may your love bless the world.

RESOURCES

- Sara Billups, *Nervous Systems: Spiritual Practices to Calm Anxiety in Your Body, the Church, and Politics*
- Tod Bolsinger, *Canoeing the Mountains: Christian Leadership in Uncharted Territory*
- Steve Cuss, *Managing Leadership Anxiety: Yours and Theirs*
- Jim Herrington, Trisha Taylor, and R. Robert Creech, *The Leader's Journey: Accepting the Call to Personal and Congregational Transformation*
- Henri J. M. Nouwen, *In the Name of Jesus: Reflections on Christian Leadership*

REFLECTION

1. Take a few minutes to journal from this prompt: How am I chasing worth, belonging, and purpose? How might this impact how I love others?
2. Take a moment to consider how enmeshment or fusion might apply to you. What story from your own life or way of relating reflects this posture? What shift did you notice in your body when you attempted to meet external expectations at the expense of your own needs? Would you consider this an outlier or typical of your relational pattern?
3. Take a moment to consider how detachment or avoidance might apply to you. What story from your own life or way of relating reflects this posture? What shift did you notice in your body when you sought distance from someone or something? Would you consider this an outlier or typical of your relational pattern?

4. Consider a time within a relationship, group, or larger system when you felt activated or triggered. Attune to the stimulation of emotion or the swirl of sensations in your body. Can you sense a connection to a younger version of yourself in that feeling? About how old do/did you feel? How might you connect with compassion to that younger you? How might you allow that feeling to awaken some curiosity about why and how you relate today?
5. Consider someone you know or have worked with whose presence feels safe and grounded. What shifts within you when you're around this person, as opposed to being around someone who is undifferentiated and dysregulated?

PRACTICE
Cultivating Loving Relationship for the Sake of Character Change

Reshaped to Love

Let's consider practices that can invite curiosity and change within you.

Consider the very first question God asks in Genesis 3:9 after Adam and Eve have grasped for external satisfaction amidst the serpent's lies. God asks, "Where are you?" This invites not just internal inquiry, but relational curiosity too. Consider a recent relational interaction you've had, and reflect on the experience with the following prompts:

- Did you show up with authenticity?
- Did you overaccommodate or avoid?
- Did you please or perform?
- Did you silence yourself or shrink?

Notice your body. Become curious about how fusion or detachment show up.

Sit quietly and recall a moment of feeling emotionally fused or overly responsible. Where did you feel it in your body? Tight chest? Nausea? Tension in the jaw?

Now do the same with a memory of shutting down or withdrawing. Where did you go numb? Did your body feel far away, disconnected?

Name and notice; write out what you observed using the following as a guide: "My chest tightens when I feel pulled to rescue. That tells me I'm leaving myself." Labeling without judgment fosters nervous system regulation.

Seeking relational feedback

To grow in differentiation, it's vital not only to explore your inner world, but to open yourself to how others experience you. This practice invites compassionate curiosity—not for self-judgment or people-pleasing, but for wholeness. When received with an open heart, the reflections of trusted people in your life can help you better understand your impact, relational style, and blind spots.

STEP 1: PREPARE YOUR HEART

Before reaching out to anyone, take a few breaths. Notice if you're seeking affirmation or if you're open to honest reflection.

Remind yourself: This is not about pleasing or performing. It's about presence and growth.

STEP 2: CHOOSE TWO TO THREE TRUSTED PEOPLE

Select individuals who know you well and whom you trust to speak honestly and kindly—perhaps a friend, partner, colleague, mentor, or trusted family member.

STEP 3: ASK WITH OPENNESS

Say, "I'm curious to know how you experience me." Follow up with these questions:

- "What do you notice about my relational style?"
- "How do I show up well or not so well, and in what contexts?"
- "Where do you see me impacting others? What does that look like? Where has it been hurtful to others?"
- "When have you seen me closed off, refusing to make an impact?"
- "How do I show up in conflict or when under stress?"
- "How might I tend to control, disappear, please, overfunction, or merge with others?"

STEP 4: RECEIVE AND REFLECT

Don't interrupt or explain. Just listen. Take notes if helpful.

Afterward, reflect:

- What resonates?
- What surprised you?
- Where did you notice defensiveness in your spirit? What might this be connected to?
- What part of you might be self-protective in these moments?

STEP 5: INTEGRATE

Take what you've learned into journaling, therapy, or prayer. Ask:

- How does this feedback align with your own experience of yourself?
- What does it reveal about your patterns of fusion or detachment?
- What small shift can you make toward deeper, more grounded presence?
- How are you being invited to love in a more authentic and wholehearted way?

a letter to you, the reader

Dear Friend,

If you've made it here, you've done something courageous.

You have not merely read a book. You have lingered over questions that many spend a lifetime avoiding. You have explored the foundation, maturation, and transformation of your character—and the character of those around you. And you have allowed yourself to consider, not just what you do, but who you are becoming.

For that, I am deeply grateful.

I've felt the gravity of these words as I've written them, not least because they touch the tender places in all of us. These are the real places in your life and mine shaped by love and loss, by failure and foolishness, by heartache and "hope deferred" (Proverbs 13:12).

This work of character transformation, I've said, is not cosmetic. It is not about behavioral tinkering, image management, or spiritual performance.

It is about the slow reordering of love.

It is about healing what has been fractured. It is about becoming whole. It is about intentional engagement that bears fruit. It is about being drawn into the very life of Christ, whose self-giving love reconciles, restores, and renews all that has been fractured.

And that is no small thing.

To Those Who Have Been Harmed

I want to speak directly, for a moment, to those who have been wounded—by a parent, a partner, a pastor, a critic, a leader, a system, a church, or someone who bore the name of Christ but not his character.

If you have read these pages wondering whether the one who hurt you will ever change, I want you to hear this clearly: *Your healing does not depend on their transformation.*

It is not naive to long for someone to change. It is human. But please do not tether your future to their willingness to do the work. You are permitted to seek safety. You are permitted to forge a life in goodness, beauty, and truth. You are permitted to step into the light of your own healing—even if they remain in the dark. You are permitted to grow—even if they do not.

And please hear this: You are permitted to grieve.

It is all right to lament what was taken from you—trust broken, years lost, reputation harmed, health impacted, body braced. It is all right to feel anger at what should never have happened. And amidst it all, it is good and right to take all the time you need to cultivate safety, healthy connection, and clarity about who you are and what your next steps will be.

To Those Who Simply Long to Grow

Perhaps you are not in crisis. Perhaps no scandal has erupted, no public failure has exposed a secret life. Perhaps you simply sense a quiet longing to be more grounded, more present, more loving, more like Jesus.

You want to be less reactive, less anxious, less defensive.

You long to be the kind of person whose presence steadies a room rather than unsettles it. The leader who does not need to dominate to feel secure. The spouse, friend, or parent whose love feels safe. The advocate whose pursuit of justice is grounded.

That longing is holy.

Maturity is not reserved for spiritual elites or therapy veterans. It is the ordinary call of every human being. We are all becoming someone. The only question is whether we are becoming that someone unconsciously—or intentionally.

The work is not glamorous. It is often hidden. And it will unfold, in time, in the small choices you make:

The pause before speaking to notice what's stirring within.
The willingness to repair after rupture.
The courage to admit, "I was wrong."
The discipline of telling yourself and others the truth when it would be easier to perform.

That you're longing for more is profoundly hopeful. I honor that longing in you—and I honor the new habits you're forming, the new choices you're making, and the life of love that is emerging within you. It might unfold more slowly than you or I would like. But it is emerging, no less. Trust that what you've started will bear fruit.

The Slow Becoming

Indeed, friends—change is slow.

We live in an age of quick fixes and curated personas. We prefer quick comebacks to costly repentance. We chase relief more than we cultivate depth.

But, as we've explored, the soul does not ripen under pressure. It ripens with patient tending. Learn to resist the urgency and rediscover a pace that's just right for you.

You may feel discouraged that you are not "further along." You may still notice your old patterns—your defensiveness, your scarcity, your need for approval, your tendency to withdraw or control. I do too.

Do not be surprised.

Formation is not linear. There are seasons of clarity and seasons of fog. There are breakthroughs and regressions. There are moments when you feel expansive and integrated—and others when you feel fragmented again.

The question is not whether you will stumble.

The question is whether you will return.

Return to honesty.
Return to curiosity about your inner world.
Return to the steady work of aligning your outer life with your inner longings.
Return to the one who knows you fully and loves you still.

Grace meets you there—not rushing you, not shaming you, but tending you toward wholeness.

A Word About Justice and Hope

Character is not merely personal. It is relational, communal, and systemic.

We are shaped in families, churches, institutions, and cultures that cultivate integrity at times and that reward performance and power at others.

To grow in character is not merely to become more kind, though the world aches for kindness. It is to become people who band with others to refuse to participate in cycles of harm. It is to become leaders who seek to protect the vulnerable. It is to be willing to help dismantle systems that protect power, fracture dignity, and distort love. It is to embody a maturity that holds both empathy and accountability—not confusing mercy with minimizing abuse or forgiveness with forced reconciliation.

Justice is not opposed to compassion. In fact, true compassion tells the truth about harm. It names coercion. It confronts control. It establishes consequences. And when necessary, it creates distance to protect those who have been wounded.

We need such people now.

We need leaders who are not dazzled by charisma but anchored in humility.
Communities that value truth over image.
Churches that care more about safe connection than reputation.
Jesus followers who walk the way of the Lamb, not the way of the sword.

If you have felt disillusioned by what you've witnessed, by all means grieve—but do not let cynicism have the final word. Let your grief metabolize into grounded trust, buttressed by resilient hope, so that you live in love as an ambassador of God's shalom in the world.

An Invitation

So where do you go from here?

You deepen.

You cultivate safety in a body that has lived under subtle threat, building connection within in a way that fosters communion and compassion.

You sink your roots and risk being known as you are, forgoing fauxnerability for an authenticity that awakens you to your true self.

You seek the right kind of attention, turning inward with curiosity, and feeling seen and soothed in a way that quiets the urgent clamoring within.

You allow safety, eldering, community, and a sacred story to hold you, so that your suffering ripens you rather than retraumatizes you.

You welcome back the parts of yourself that once felt fragmented, growing more whole not through strategies of suppression but steps toward self-compassion.

You awaken to the season of the journey you are in, with its unique challenges and tasks for your maturation.

You anchor your faith in something deeper than fear, fight, or the urge to fix.

You imagine hope that does not deny pain but grows more resilient.

And at last, you embody love—steady enough to remain present in anxious and avoidant systems, courageous enough to move toward others without losing yourself.

In the process of becoming who you are, you'll see—slowly, almost imperceptibly—your life begin to overflow with the relational fruit of love, joy, peace, patience, kindness, goodness, faithfulness, gentleness, and self-control.

And when you disappoint yourself and others—*and you will*—you'll start to notice something else. You'll refuse shame's lie that nothing has changed. You'll notice what has happened and begin again.

This is slow and courageous work.

But you are not alone in it. I'm with you in it—and there are many others who hunger and thirst for so much more.

And so, dear friends, let this final blessing linger with you as you step into your own becoming, rooted and grounded in God's love:

May you feel regulated and steadied in a world that thrives on agitation,
safe in your own body and a safe presence to others.

May you be rooted beneath performance,
free to be known without pretending.

May you grow more reflective,
attentive to what shapes you and soothes you.

May your suffering ripen you rather than render you bitter,
growing you into a person of wisdom who can elder others along the way.

May what has been fragmented in you be reintegrated,
so that integrity manifests in wholehearted presence.

May your loves be reoriented,
your ambitions surrendered to a deeper call.

May your faith be renewed,
grounded enough to resist fear and free enough to relinquish the need to fight or fix.

May your hope be resilient,
tender enough to feel the wound and strong enough to remain open in its presence.

May your life be relational,
secure enough to move toward others without losing yourself and generous enough to embody self-giving love.

Slowly, by grace,
may you become who you have always been in the heart of God.

And may the life you live—quietly, consistently—become a testimony not to your perfection, but to your slow and patient maturation.

With gratitude and hope,
Chuck

acknowledgments

Most of this book was written in a black West Elm recliner that sits in the living room of our small mid-century modern home in Grand Rapids. The chair has held me for many early mornings, the quiet hours when the house is still and the big living room windows frame Michigan's widely divergent seasons—some days buried in feet of winter snow, other days warmed by a rising sun that gradually fills the room with light.

From that chair I can see the table where our family gathers when we're all home. That happens less often these days. Both of our daughters are married now, and the rhythms of life have shifted in beautiful ways. But when I look across the room at that table, I'm reminded why writing a book on character feels both important and a little daunting.

Because the people who sit around that table know me best.

They are the ones most affected by my character. They know my contradictions, and they've seen the places where my words and my life do not always align. Writing a book about character while being known that deeply is a vulnerable thing.

And yet, by the mysterious grace of God, this home has been a safe place for all of us. It is a place where laughter has often been louder than our disagreements, where tears have been shed without shame, and where truth—sometimes difficult truth—has been spoken. It is a place where grace has slowly done its quiet work.

Most mornings, I worked on this book before the house fully woke. At some point Sara would quietly walk into the kitchen to make her first cup of coffee. That simple movement—her gentle presence entering the room—was always a quiet reassurance. Sara has been the steady ground beneath so much of my life and work. Thank you, Sara, for your patience, your encouragement, and your secure love. I'm grateful that in this season of our lives we're able to slow down a bit, dream together, and find ourselves traveling to places of beauty and peace.

Soon enough, my younger daughter, Maggie, would rise as well. During much of this writing she was still living with us, often busy with wedding planning, which meant I had the joy of watching the simple, everyday delight she took in carefully stewarding the details of that special day, often with Sara right by her side. And every other weekend Micah would come to stay with us, which meant I had the gift of seeing their relationship up close: the easy connection between them, the deep faithfulness they share, and the genuine delight they take in one another. Maggie and Micah, watching the two of you together is like witnessing a living picture of love, joy, peace, patience, kindness, and gentle faithfulness that sustain a shared life.

Most weekdays I'd eventually make my way over to the seminary, where my older daughter, Emma, and her husband, Sam, are students in the clinical mental health counseling program I have the privilege of stewarding. Sam and Emma, it has been a deep joy to watch the two of you mature in marriage and grow into your gifts. Emma, you carry a warmth that seems to fill the hallways and classrooms with life—your smile alone can lift my spirits and lighten the day. And Sam, you bring a thoughtful curiosity and the kind of deep questions that invite everyone around you to think more carefully and live more honestly. You were always the first to ask about the progress of this book and the most eager to devour the manuscript once it was finished. What I admire most about the two of you is the way you refuse to hide your imperfections or smooth over your inconsistencies, modeling a courageous vulnerability that invites the rest of us to live more honestly too.

As I wrote these pages, I thought often about my mom and dad, both of whom passed away over the last couple of years. I've spoken candidly about parts of our story in my writing over the years, including some of their shortcomings. But what brings me deep comfort now is remembering the heartfelt conversations we shared too—conversations that reshaped our relationship. Though I didn't always know it earlier in life, those moments reminded me that they did, in their own ways, love the person I had become. I am grateful for that.

Beyond the circle of our home, there are others who have quietly shaped this book's journey—dear friends and colleagues. Like Ryan, whose frequent and earnest check-ins felt like air when I was suffocating. And Kyle, whose faithful friendship over fifteen years steadies me. And Elizabeth, a dear friend who profoundly models both humility and integrity, and whose hard work enabled us to create the clinical mental health counseling program at Western Theological Seminary. And there are so many others, professionally and personally, who see me, support me, and say hard things to me too.

About five years ago I began searching for an agent and publisher who valued connection, integrity, honesty, and open communication—and in that search I found not just professional partners, but friendships.

My agent, Don Gates, carries the rare combination of affirming the deep value of a writer's work while also offering the kind of honest and compassionate feedback that helps it become stronger. Don, you have the rare gift of supporting both the vision and the craft of a book, and I am grateful for your wisdom and partnership.

At Tyndale, Jillian Schlossberg has once again shepherded this manuscript with extraordinary care. Jillian has a remarkable capacity to listen deeply to an author's voice while also asking the kinds of questions that clarify and strengthen the work. Jillian, your guidance has made this book better in ways readers may never see but will certainly feel.

And Kim Miller, whose attentive editing shaped sentences, paragraphs, and entire sections with such skill and discernment. Kim, you've known how to encourage me and challenge me. I'm deeply grateful for your careful and compassionate work.

And to Dean Renninger, Brandi Davis, Elise Peterson, Brittany Buczynski, Brianna Coyle, Megan D'Agostino, Stephanie Abrassart, and Zoe Jethani at Tyndale, for the quiet, faith-filled, behind-the-scenes companionship that doesn't seek the spotlight but faithfully supports the work.

Much of this book was written while being held by that black West Elm recliner in our living room. But more truly, I have been held by the God who, as St. Patrick's ancient prayer recalls, is with me and within me, before me and behind me, above me and beneath me, to my right and to my left—ripening me all the while. May God grow us, mature us, and ripen us with grace—lifting us when we fall and filling our lives with love and enduring hope.

notes

INTRODUCTION: CAN I TRUST YOU?

1. *Abuse and Psychological Coercion: An Investigation into Thomas Philippe, Jean Vanier and L'Arche*, Summary of the Study Commission's report mandated by L'Arche International (January 2023), 31, 49, https://commissiondetude-jeanvanier.org/commissiondetudeindependante2023-empriseetabus/wp-content/uploads/2023/03/Summary-Study-Commission-Report-EN_March2023.pdf.
2. Phyllis Tickle, *The Great Emergence: How Christianity Is Changing and Why* (Baker Books, 2008), 16.
3. Jonathan T. Pennington, *The Sermon on the Mount and Human Flourishing: A Theological Commentary* (Baker Academic, 2017).
4. "Psalms of Complaint—Study Guide," Yale Bible Study, accessed February 27, 2026, https://yalebiblestudy.org/courses/psalms/lessons/psalms-of-complaint-study-guide/. See a similar lament reflection in my book *Healing What's Within* (Tyndale Refresh, 2024), 50.

CHAPTER 1: REGULATED

1. James K. A. Smith, *You Are What You Love: The Spiritual Power of Habit* (Baker, 2016), 36.
2. Rowan Williams, *Passions of the Soul* (Bloomsbury, 2024), xxiii.
3. For more on the internal hyper- and hypoarousal states that I refer to as Storm and Fog, see my book *Healing What's Within*, 60–67.
4. See Daniel Siegel and Mary Hartzell's *Parenting from the Inside Out* (Tarcher, 2003) for their tips on what they call "good enough parenting."
5. For more on these dynamics, see Aimie Apigian, *The Biology of Trauma* (BenBella Books, 2025).

6. For more on understanding this spectrum and how I assess folks, see my book *When Narcissism Comes to Church: Healing Your Community from Emotional and Spiritual Abuse* (InterVarsity Press, 2020).
7. Dallas Willard, *The Divine Conspiracy: Rediscovering Our Hidden Life in God* (HarperOne, 1998), 41.
8. Smith, *You Are What You Love*, 10.
9. Thomas Chalmers, *The Expulsive Power of a New Affection* (Crossway, 2020).
10. Williams, *Passions of the Soul*, xxv.
11. For more on these four S's, see Daniel J. Siegel and Tina Payne Bryson, *The Power of Showing Up: How Parental Presence Shapes Who Our Kids Become and How Their Brains Get Wired* (Ballantine Books, 2020).

CHAPTER 2: ROOTED

1. Gabor Maté, *The Myth of Normal: Trauma, Illness, and Healing in a Toxic Culture* (Penguin Random House, 2022), 106–107.
2. For more on *inscape* and *haecceitas*, see Daniel P. Horan, *The Franciscan Heart of Thomas Merton: A New Look at the Spiritual Inspiration of His Life, Thought, and Writing* (Ave Maria Press, 2013).
3. See Carl Gustav Jung, *The Development of Personality*, trans. R. F. C. Hull, vol. 17 of *The Collected Works of C. G. Jung*, 2nd ed. (Princeton University Press, 1954).
4. This isn't at all to minimize the importance of psychotropic medications, which I've personally found great benefit in, but to point out how curiosity about the deeper realities within can be even more helpful.
5. Thomas Merton, *Choosing to Love the World: On Contemplation* (Sounds True, 2008), 30.
6. Wayne King, "Swaggart Says He Has Sinned; Will Step Down," *New York Times*, February 22, 1988, https://www.nytimes.com/1988/02/22/us/swaggart-says-he-has-sinned-will-step-down.html; Peter H. King, "'What's Past Is Past': A Defiant Swaggart Returns to the Pulpit," *Los Angeles Times*, May 23, 1988, https://www.latimes.com/archives/la-xpm-1988-05-23-mn-2141-story.html.
7. Mary Oliver, "The Journey," in *Dream Work* (Atlantic Monthly Press, 1986), 38.
8. Augustine of Hippo, *Expositions of the Psalms 121–150*, ed. Boniface Ramsey, trans. Boniface Ramsey and Maria Boulding, vol. 20 of *The Works of Saint Augustine* (New City Press, 2004), 404.
9. Curt Thompson, *The Soul of Shame: Retelling the Stories We Believe About Ourselves* (InterVarsity Press, 2015), 138.

CHAPTER 3: REFLECTIVE

1. Wesley Granberg-Michaelson, "Pay Attention to Where You Pay Attention," *The Soulwork of Justice*, Substack, July 24, 2025, https://wesgm.substack.com/p/pay-atttention-to-where-you-pay-attention.

2. *The Screwtape Letters* (HarperOne, 1942) is a satirical look at the many ways humans are tempted, as revealed in an exchange of letters between the fictional senior devil, Screwtape, and his inexperienced nephew, Wormwood.
3. Anna Lembke, *Dopamine Nation: Finding Balance in the Age of Indulgence* (Dutton, 2021).
4. James Clear, *Atomic Habits: An Easy and Proven Way to Build Good Habits and Break Bad Ones* (Avery, 2018), 201.
5. Joe Dispenza, *You Are the Placebo: Making Your Mind Matter* (Hay House Publishing, 2014), 51.
6. Mary Oliver, *Upstream* (Penguin, 2016), 7.
7. Curt Thompson, *Anatomy of the Soul: Surprising Connections Between Neuroscience and Spiritual Practices That Can Transform Your Life and Relationships* (Tyndale Refresh, 2010), 52.
8. I've heard a variation of this phrase from the philosophers James K. A. Smith and Marshall McLuhan.
9. Steven Garber, *The Fabric of Faithfulness: Weaving Together Belief and Behavior During the University Years* (InterVarsity Press, 1996), 56.
10. N. T. Wright, *After You Believe: Why Christian Character Matters* (HarperOne, 2010), 20–21.
11. Fyodor Dostoevsky, *The Brothers Karamazov*, trans. Constance Garnett (Macmillan, 1922), 66–67.
12. C. S. Lewis, *Mere Christianity* (Touchstone, 1996), 147.
13. C. S. Lewis, *The Screwtape Letters* (HarperCollins, 1996), 59, 60.
14. Augustine, *Confessions*, trans. Henry Chadwick (Oxford University Press, 2008), 201.

CHAPTER 4: RIPENED

1. Walter Brueggemann, *The Psalms and the Life of Faith*, ed. Patrick D. Miller (Fortress, 1995), 67–68.
2. Frederick Buechner, "The Stewardship of Pain," *30 Good Minutes*, The Chicago Sunday Evening Club, 4:35, aired January 27, 1991, youtube.com/watch?v=73hdH1_z2ps.
3. Michael Gurian, *Mothers, Sons, and Lovers: How a Man's Relationship with His Mother Affects the Rest of His Life* (Shambhala, 1994), 30.
4. David G. Gilmore, *Manhood in the Making: Cultural Concepts of Masculinity* (Yale University Press, 1990).
5. Christy Angelle Bauman, *Her Rites: A Sacred Journey for the Mind, Body, and Soul* (Convergent, 2024).
6. Etty Hillesum, *Etty Hillesum: An Interrupted Life: the Diaries, 1941–1943; and Letters from Westerbork*, trans. Arnold J. Pomerans (Metropolitan, 1996), 96–97.

7. Hillesum, *Etty Hillesum: An Interrupted Life*, 44, 178.
8. For more information on the story workshops offered by the Allender Center, see https://theallendercenter.org/offerings/workshops/the-story-workshop/.
9. Examples in Christian spaces include initiatory pathways like Jon Tyson's Primal Path, Rusty McKie's ManSchool, and Christy Bauman's Womaneering retreats. Other formational spaces include The Soul Care Institute, Anam Cara Ministries, the KINEO Center, and the New Life Fellowship School of Formation. Beyond explicitly Christian spaces, you'll find the work of Clarissa Pinkola Estés, Sacred Sons, Richard Rohr's Men's Rites of Passage, Hillary McBride and Lisa Gungor's Sacred Feminine retreats, Red Tent Gatherings, and Francis Weller's grief work. But this is just a small sampling.
10. See especially authors like Cole Arthur Riley and Karen Gonzalez who write in this vein, or see a formational experience like Peter Choi's Center for Faith and Justice.
11. See the work of The Porter's Gate worship project at https://www.portersgateworship.com/.
12. Cole Arthur Riley, *This Here Flesh: Spirituality, Liberation, and the Stories That Make Us* (Convergent, 2022), 98–99.

CHAPTER 5: REINTEGRATED

1. See Chuck DeGroat, *Wholeheartedness: Busyness, Exhaustion, and Healing the Divided Self* (Eerdmans, 2016).
2. Augustine of Hippo, *Expositions of the Psalms 121–150*, ed. Boniface Ramsey, trans. Boniface Ramsey and Maria Boulding, vol. 20 of *The Works of Saint Augustine* (New City Press, 2004), 469.
3. Evagrius Ponticus, *The Praktikos and Chapters on Prayer*, trans. John Eudes Bamberger (Cistercian Publications, 1972), 18.
4. Parker J. Palmer, *Let Your Life Speak: Listening for the Voice of Vocation* (Jossey-Bass, 2000), 12.
5. James Baldwin, "As Much Truth As One Can Bear," *The New York Times Book Review*, January 14, 1962, BR38.
6. This short video from the BibleProject is helpful: https://bibleproject.com/videos/vocab-insight-teleios-whole/.
7. Mechthild of Magdeburg, *The Flowing Light of the Godhead*, trans. Frank Tobin (Paulist Press, 1998), Book IV, §2.
8. Søren Kierkegaard, *Purity of Heart Is to Will One Thing: Spiritual Preparation for the Office of Confession*, trans. Douglas V. Steere (Harper & Row, 1956).
9. See my book *Wholeheartedness: Busyness, Exhaustion, and Healing the Divided Self* (Eerdmans, 2016).

CHAPTER 6: REORIENTED

1. U2, "Stuck in a Moment You Can't Get Out Of" by Paul David Hewson, Adam Clayton, Larry Mullen, and David Howell Evans, on *All That You Can't Leave Behind,* Island Records, 2000, compact disc.
2. Bruce Demarest, "Reflections on Developmental Spirituality: Journey Paradigms and Stages," *Journal of Spiritual Formation and Soul Care* 1, no. 2 (2008): 149–167.
3. See Psalm 1:3; Job 12:12; and John 15:2.
4. Erik H. Erikson, *The Life Cycle Completed* (W. W. Norton, 1982).
5. James W. Fowler, *Stages of Faith: The Psychology of Human Development and the Quest for Meaning* (Harper, 1981).
6. Mary Oliver, "Have You Ever Tried to Enter the Long Black Branches," in *West Wind: Poems and Prose Poems* (Houghton Mifflin, 1997), 140.
7. Irenaeus, *Against Heresies*, 4.11.2; *Ante-Nicene Fathers*, volume 1 (Eerdmans, 1979), 474.
8. Walter Brueggemann, *The Psalms and the Life of Faith* (Fortress Press, 1995), 9.
9. See also Brian Purfield, "Reading the Old Testament," London Jesuit Centre, February 2021, 14.
10. For example, in the twelfth century, St. Bernard of Clairvaux offered a four-fold path, describing the spiritual life as a journey of love. The fourteenth-century Flemish mystic Jan van Ruusbroec framed the spiritual journey in three interwoven movements: the active life, the interior life, and the contemplative life. Two centuries later, St. John of the Cross described four stages of deepening maturation and union in the journey of faith.
11. For more, see Chuck DeGroat, *Wild Country of the Heart: Navigating the Seasons of the Spiritual Journey with St. Teresa of Ávila* film and study guide, accessed July 16, 2025, chuckdegroat.net/wild-country-of-the-heart.
12. Teresa of Ávila, *The Interior Castle*, trans. Mirabai Starr (Riverhead, 2003), 35.
13. Samuel Trevor Francis, "O the Deep, Deep Love of Jesus!," 1875, https://hymnallibrary.org/hymns/o-the-deep-deep-love-of-jesus/.
14. Teresa of Ávila, *The Interior Castle*, 57.
15. Teresa of Ávila, *The Interior Castle*, 77.
16. Janet Hagberg and Robert Guelich, *The Critical Journey* (Sheffield Press, 1995), 232.
17. Cornelius Plantinga Jr., *Not the Way It's Supposed to Be: A Breviary of Sin* (Eerdmans, 1995), 34–35.
18. Mary Oliver, *Upstream: Selected Essays* (Penguin Press, 2016), 3–4.

CHAPTER 7: RENEWED

1. Iain McGilchrist, *The Master and His Emissary: The Divided Brain and the Making of the Western World* (Yale University Press, 2009).

2. See Curt Thompson, *Anatomy of the Soul: Surprising Connections Between Neuroscience and Spiritual Practices That Can Transform Your Life and Relationships* (Tyndale Refresh, 2010).
3. Lesslie Newbigin writes about "proper confidence" in his book by the same name. It is a confidence that is neither absolutist nor relativistic, locating conviction within humility, communal discernment, and ongoing openness to correction. See Lesslie Newbigin, *Proper Confidence: Faith, Doubt, and Certainty in Christian Discipleship* (Eerdmans, 1995).

CHAPTER 8: RESILIENT

1. Kelly Clarkson, vocalist, "Stronger (What Doesn't Kill You)," by Jörgen Elofsson, Ali Tamposi, David Gamson, and Greg Kurstin, track 2 on *Stronger*, RCA, 2011.
2. Eugene H. Peterson, *A Long Obedience in the Same Direction: Discipleship in an Instant Society* (InterVarsity Press, 1980).
3. *The Shawshank Redemption*, written and directed by Frank Darabont (Warner Bros., 1994), film.
4. *The Lord of the Rings: The Two Towers*, directed by Peter Jackson, screenplay by Fran Walsh, Peter Jackson, Stephen Sinclair, and Philippa Boyens, based on the novel by J. R. R. Tolkien (New Line Cinema, 2002), DVD.
5. One of my favorite resources on the application of neuroplasticity is Bonnie Badenoch, *Being a Brain-Wise Therapist: A Practical Guide to Interpersonal Neurobiology* (W. W. Norton, 2008).
6. See Daniel J. Siegel, *The Mindful Brain: Reflection and Attunement in the Cultivation of Well-Being* (W. W. Norton, 2007).
7. Teresa of Ávila, *The Interior Castle*, trans. Mirabai Starr (Riverhead Books, 2003), 42–43.
8. Francis de Sales, *Introduction to the Devout Life*, trans. John K. Ryan (New York: Image Books, 1972), 60–61.
9. On this theme, see Aundi Kolber, *Try Softer: A Fresh Approach to Move Us out of Anxiety, Stress, and Survival Mode—and into a Life of Connection and Joy* (Tyndale Momentum, 2020).
10. See chapters 1–3 in my book *Healing What's Within.*
11. Some resources on retraining the brain that I discovered include Jeffrey M. Schwartz and Rebecca Gladding, *You Are Not Your Brain: The 4-Step Solution for Changing Bad Habits, Ending Unhealthy Thinking, and Taking Control of Your Life* (Avery, 2011); Lisa Wimberger, *Neurosculpting: A Whole-Brain Approach to Heal Trauma, Rewrite Limiting Beliefs, and Find Wholeness* (Sounds True, 2015); Annie Hopper, *Wired for Healing: Remapping the Brain to Recover from Chronic and Mysterious Illnesses* (DNRS Publishing, 2014); and Joe Dispenza, *Breaking the*

Habit of Being Yourself: How to Lose Your Mind and Create a New One (Hay House, 2012).

12. Neural retraining is a practice developed by Annie Hopper and explored in her book *Wired for Healing*.
13. Researcher and chiropractor Joe Dispenza expands on this in his book *Breaking the Habit of Being Yourself*.
14. "Read Martin Luther King Jr.'s 'I Have a Dream' Speech in Its Entirety," WBEZ Chicago, January 16, 2023, https://www.npr.org/2010/01/18/122701268/i-have-a-dream-speech-in-its-entirety.
15. Joe Dispenza developed this process of visualization and mental rehearsal to imagine his body's healing process after devastating triathlon injuries.

CHAPTER 9: RELATIONAL

1. James Bartholomew, "The Awful Rise of 'Virtue Signalling,'" *The Spectator*, April 18, 2015, https://www.spectator.co.uk/article/the-awful-rise-of-virtue-signalling/.
2. Murray Bowen, *Family Therapy in Clinical Practice* (Rowman and Littlefield, 1993).
3. On this, see my book *Healing What's Within: Coming Home to Yourself—and to God—When You're Wounded, Weary, and Wandering* (Tyndale Refresh, 2024).
4. Pete Scazzero, "Skills to Revolutionize Your Prayer Life Pt. 2: Climb the Ladder," *Emotionally Healthy Leader Podcast*, March 9, 2021, https://www.emotionallyhealthy.org/podcast/detail/Skills-to-Revolutionize-Your-Prayer-Life-Pt.-2-Climb-the-Ladder/.
5. Walter Bauer, William F. Arndt, and F. Wilbur Gingrich, *A Greek-English Lexicon of the New Testament and Other Early Christian Literature*, ed. Frederick William Danker, 3rd ed. (University of Chicago Press, 2000), s.v. "σπλαγχνίζομαι."
6. See Paul Bloom, *Against Empathy: The Case for Rational Compassion* (HarperCollins, 2016) and Joe Rigney, *The Sin of Empathy: Compassion and Its Counterfeits* (Canon Press, 2025).
7. For a contemporary history of empathy, see Susan Lanzoni, *Empathy: A History* (Yale University Press, 2018).
8. "Empathy Fatigue: How Stress and Trauma Can Take a Toll on You," Cleveland Clinic, last modified April 14, 2022, https://health.clevelandclinic.org/empathy-fatigue-how-stress-and-trauma-can-take-a-toll-on-you.
9. Henri J. M. Nouwen, *Reaching Out: The Three Movements of the Spiritual Life* (Image, 1986), 32.

about the author

Chuck DeGroat is a professor of pastoral care and Christian spirituality at Western Theological Seminary in Holland, Michigan, where he also serves as founding executive director of the clinical mental health counseling program. He is a licensed therapist, spiritual director, author, retreat leader, and founder of The Soul Care Collaborative, a network of practitioners offering spiritually attuned and trauma-informed care. As a therapist, he specializes in navigating issues of abuse and trauma, pastoral (and leadership) health, and doubt and dark nights on the faith journey. He and his team also facilitate five-day soul care intensives. He trains clergy in handling issues of abuse and trauma, and he conducts pastor and planter assessments. Before transitioning to training and forming pastors, Chuck served as a pastor and counseling center director in Orlando and San Francisco. He and his wife, Sara, have two married daughters. Visit Chuck online at chuckdegroat.net and soulcarecollaborative.com.